SEX TIPS
for
GIRLS

by
Cynthia Heimel

A FIRESIDE BOOK
Published by Simon & Schuster Inc.
New York London Toronto Sydney Tokyo Singapore

First Fireside Edition, 1986

Published by Simon & Schuster Inc.
Simon & Schuster Building
Rockefeller Center
1230 Avenue of the Americas
New York, New York 10020

FIRESIDE and colophon are registered trademarks of Simon &
Schuster, Inc. Manufactured in the United States of America

10 9 8 7 6 5 4 3 2

Pbk. 10 9 8 7

Library of Congress Cataloging in Publication Data

Heimel, Cynthia, date.
    Sex tips for girls.

    1. Sex—Anecdotes, facetiae, satire, etc.
I. Title.
PN6231.S54H44   1983   818'.5402   83-509
ISBN 0-671-44997-4
ISBN 0-671-47725-0 Pbk.

Portions of this book have appeared in slightly different form in *New
York Magazine* and the *Village Voice*.

"Faded Love" by John Wills, Bob Wills, copyright © 1950, 1951 by Bob
Wills Music, Inc. Copyrights renewed, assigned to Unichappell Music,
Inc. (Rightsong Music, Publisher).

THIS BOOK IS DEDICATED TO
MARY PEACOCK, SARAH LONGACRE, AND GINGER VARNEY.

Acknowledgments

Almost everyone I've ever met has helped me, directly or indirectly, with this book. But in a few cases the help was so supreme that I must name names.

The first person I must thank is my son Brodie, an angel with a catcher's mitt and clarinet, who brought me cheeseburgers when I needed them most. Heartfelt thanks also to my editor, Patricia Soliman, and my agent, Ron Bernstein, without whom I would be a basket case.

I am eternally grateful to my friends who consented to have their brains picked. The girls: Nancy Cardozo, Lynne Geller, Leslye Noyes, Maggie Wood, Jennifer Thompson, Emily Prager, Annie Flanders, Chris Kapp, Marcia Resnick, Carol Troy, Pucci Meyer, Andrea Port, Carol Leggett, and Joyce Korn. The boys: Stephen Saban, Lewis Grossberger, Mark Jacobson, David Silver, Danny Goldberg, Robert Younger, John Prine, Big Boy Medlin, Rex Weiner, John Berendt, Mick Farren, Peter Wood, and most especially, Michael Longacre.

For special services rendered I want to thank Sarah Sender, Janice and Raul G'Acha, Phil and Mary Keenan, Diane Mitchell, Steven Adcock, Philip Kingsley, David a.k.a. Harry King, Ed Kosner, and Walter Matthau.

And love to my family, who had no choice but to put up with me: Barb, Joe, Jane, Arthur, Connie, Chris, Delsa, Tim, Paul, Steve. My sister Donna, and Scott. Nanny. Mom and Dad.

Contents

1

Who Are We?

These are the times that try a girl's soul. We don't know where to turn, what to think. We lie in bed in the morning, trying to determine a good reason to get up. We often wonder whether we're in the mood for a sandwich or not.

Should we take vitamins? Wear dresses? Shave our legs? Demonstrate against nuclear power? Dance until dawn? Eat natural foods? Search for rich husbands? Take a course in French? Become diamond smugglers?

Questions cavort in our heads. Crossroads are everywhere. We don't know who we are anymore, not the way we used to.

In the '20s we were flappers. We did the Charleston and smoked furtive cigarettes and bobbed our hair. We had plenty of beaux, all of whom wore center parts and drank gin.

In the '30s we were relentlessly cheerful in the face of adversity, trying not to mind that when the stock market crashed, Daddy lost the mansion and jumped out the window. We became typists and thought ourselves lucky.

In the '40s we were willowy and brave, wearing shoulder pads while we kissed our uniformed men goodbye. Every day we went to factories and filled bullets with gunpowder, every night we sent tender love letters overseas.

In the '50s we were pert young housewives sending our gray-flannel-suited husbands to the rat race every morning with square breakfasts in their bellies. We bought all the latest products and wore snazzy cocktail dresses to entertain hubby's boss on our Japanese-lantern-strung patios.

In the '60s we let our hair grow and fell in love with rock musicians and smoked grass and didn't mind our boyfriends' sleeping with everyone in sight. Because we were cool. We took the pill or breastfed our babies and tied silly tie-dyed bands around our heads.

In the '70s we sought to find ourselves. We hated men and decided to live alone and have a fabulously remunerative career. We joined consciousness-raising groups and became feminists. No one was allowed to light our cigarettes for us without getting a karate chop to the neck. We decided not to have children and to find our own space instead.

But now what? Whither us? We no longer have role models or prescribed modes of behavior.

Some will blame our current confusion on the alleged collapse of feminism. Feminism is far, far from dead, but it is true that the movement has lost some of its zip. It was breezing along fine there for a while, with everyone all optimistic and fervent and charging around opening day-care centers, but things have undoubtedly slackened. Women seem scared and don't know where to look for guidance, since it seems as if all the leaders of the feminist movement have retreated into their individual lairs, emerging only at infrequent intervals to snarl.

Very upsetting, but we mustn't blame our erstwhile leaders. They're tired. They've been slogging away for years and are sick of being called strident bull-dykes. Who can blame them for being out of sorts?

So now it's up to us. We must shoulder the burdens of humanity and set the world straight on course. We must look snappy. But how?

The first thing a right-minded girl must do, if only for a second, is take a look around her. It will be a grisly moment, but be brave.

Things have gone all weird in the world. Those who should know better are using words like "interface" and "networking." Men who look like perfectly normal citizens are running around in ill-fitting polyester suits and polluting rivers. Women who should know better appear in gold-lamé knickers or try to close down abortion clinics. Nobody can get a decent job, a good cigar, or a sane boyfriend. You can't tell a Buick from a Chrysler. Most of the rock-and-roll played on the radio is by dead people. The universe is expanding. Movie stars run tame in the White House.

"When the going gets weird, the weird turn pro," Hunter Thompson once said in a moment of blinding clarity.

There is only one way to set the world straight. A desperate measure, but it just might work. *We must eschew anything trivial. We must embrace all that is frivolous.*

Do not confuse the two or disastrous results may ensue. Trivial things take up all your time and dull your senses, whereas frivolity is meaningful, profound, worth living and dying for. It's easy to tell the difference. All things trivial are objects, and all things frivolous are actions.

Things trivial:
Cuisinarts
Tax shelters
Committees
Life insurance
Dress shields
Encounter groups
Home computer systems
MX missiles
Conceptual art
Nouvelle cuisine
International politics
EST
Business suits
Volvo station wagons
Mortgages
Designer sunglasses

Things frivolous:
Dancing
Eating raspberries
Driving in convertibles
Drinking champagne
Kissing
Telling jokes
Planting tomatoes
Lying on the beach
Fucking
Talking on the telephone
Singing
Buying dresses

If we devote our lives to frivolity, the world will become a far, far better place. Humanity will be better able to fulfill its primary goal, that of having a good time. The struggle will be hard and uphill, but we must stand firm, take command, brook no nonsense. Damn the torpedoes, full speed ahead.

Here are a few things we must do:

1. *Have adventures.* Whenever possible, we must opt for the unknown. We do not necessarily have to hightail it over to a struggling South American country and offer our services to guerrillas hiding in the hills, but we should never turn down a trip to Madagascar just because we don't have the right outfit.

Think how it will look, fifty years from now, when our grandchildren are clamoring about our knees demanding stories of our girlhoods, if all we have to tell them is what a great moment it was when Elizabeth Taylor made a guest appearance on "General Hospital."

It will be much more gripping if we have things to say like "Well, yes, I suppose wrestling alligators for a living was somewhat exciting, but I always preferred being a nightclub proprietor in Morocco. Of course I perpetually had to watch out for drug smugglers hiding under the bed, not to mention the time when my machine gun went off by accident, but . . ."

2. *Give fear exceedingly short shrift.* God protects drunks, infants, and feisty girls, girls who are up for anything.

3. *Shun boredom.* We must quit dull jobs, leave tedious boy-friends. We will be fine, since nature abhors a vacuum.

4. *Cultivate a deviant attitude.* Unless we're vigilant, we could turn into zombies. Seedpods are furtively placed into our bedrooms while we sleep, and the next thing we know, we're craving feminine-hygiene deodorant and Hamburger Helper. This kind of behavior is called, funnily enough, normal.

A nondeviant listens to what people say and believes them. If a nondeviant is told that the world is, as it turns out, flat, she will look puzzled for a moment, but then she will shrug her shoulders and say, "Oh, really? Fancy that."

Whereas the deviant realizes that life is short and she must be prepared to try anything.

Christopher Columbus was the first deviant. He had a fresh, un-cluttered, devil-may-care outlook. He didn't let anybody push him around, and laughed lightly when silly old stick-in-the-muds warned him he would fall off the edge of the earth. Copernicus was a de-viant, ditto da Vinci, Madame Curie, George Washington and Susan B. Anthony. All the best people, in fact.

5. *No power politics, no back-stabbing.* A lot of rubbish has been bandied about these days about looking out for number one, or número uno. Some of us take this philosophy too far, and feel per-fectly justified in ruthlessly clawing our way to the top, not minding how many innocent girls' heads we step on in our ascent.

This attitude will get us nowhere and is bad for business. Tales of our transgressions will fly around town like wildfire, since people love to talk. Before we know it, acquaintances will shun us on the street, doormen won't let us into nightclubs, even numbers runners will stroll past us with unseeing eyes.

6. *Only drink and take drugs if we have to.* It is true that William Blake said that "The Road to excess leads to the palace of wisdom," but they didn't have angel dust back then.

Sometimes it is necessary to take a Valium before reading the morning paper, or to consume a bottle of Wild Turkey if we happen to hear any version of "Send In the Clowns."

But no heavy samplings of tranquilizers designed for elephants, horses or cats if we want to wake up the next morning. No random ingesting of untested psychedelics. If we take some weird acid one minute, the next minute we could find ourselves devoting our lives to the Grateful Dead.

7. *Give sex the respect it deserves.* There are those, I will name no names, who have been trying to take sex out of the realm of the frivolous and put it into the realm of the trivial. The discoverers of the G-spot, for example. Those who go to singles bars and pick up men wearing medallions who they don't even like. Those who think romance is dead. Romance is not dead! Sex is important! Sex is profound! Sex is funny!

8. *Have another look at men.* Remember the '60s, when the battle lines were firmly drawn between hippies and law-abiding citizens? When everyone who had long hair and love beads hated everyone with short hair and business suits? You can't do that anymore, since some long-haired hippie types now build nuclear submarines (this is not a lie, I met one in Rhode Island) and some short-haired, business-suited creatures are actually lead singers in rock-and-roll bands.

During the feminist revolution, the battle lines were again simple. It was easy to tell the enemy, he was the one with the penis.

This is no longer strictly true. Some men are okay now. We're allowed to like them again. We still have to keep them in line, of course, but we no longer have to shoot them on sight.

For more about sex, men, and having a good time, please turn to the rest of this book.

2

The Great Boyfriend Crunch

MY DAY

11:30 A.M. Wake up. Realize I don't have a boyfriend. Go back to sleep again.
12:45 P.M. Wake up. Realize I don't have a boyfriend but do have intense need for sustenance. Stagger into kitchen. Make coffee. Run mind over assorted boyfriend possibilities.
1:07 P.M. Greta calling from office. She went to party last night, met cute guy. Twenty years old, too young. Also has girlfriend, but may be breaking up with her soon. We discuss possibility of starting a newsletter announcing up-to-the-second status of all heterosexual relationships in Manhattan. Girls, we figure, would line up outside office on night of publication, waiting for first copies. We would clean up. Then decide feasibility is limited—too much legwork, too depressing.

But we digress. Back to cute guy last night. We decide she should call him. Then decide she shouldn't call him, fuck him, who needs him, he has a girlfriend. Then decide she should wait a few days.

Then call. Maybe. I discuss being lonely. She discusses being lonelier. We decide we're irretrievably neurotic. Father-fixated at least. 2:13 P.M. Call Amanda. Complain about being lonely, depressed, sex-starved. Amanda interrupts to tell amusing anecdote about guy who's in love with her. He sent engagement ring—by messenger. She hates him, thinks he's a self-involved wimp. Then she immediately wonders if she has fear of intimacy. Then I wonder if I have fear of intimacy. Decide we both do. Decide to step up therapy so we can have boyfriends.

2:58 P.M. Hang up. Shower, dress, go out for breakfast. At corner restaurant see cute guy and give him come-hither glance. He pays no attention, is reading *Power! How to Get It, How to Use It.*

3:16 P.M. Home. Check answering machine for messages. Five calls. Three editors, wondering where the hell copy. Frantic message from Chris, cheery message from Cleo.

3:20 P.M. Call all editors and lie shamelessly. Then call Chris. She says husband (of ten years) is having affair, she can tell. Evidence? He disappears every afternoon, then comes home and takes shower. What's wrong with her? she wonders. Decides she has "fear of success" relationshipwise. I remind her of the ten years. She's not convinced, decides she needs shrink.

4:10 P.M. Call Cleo back. She's excited, has a date tonight. Cute guy, has job and everything.

4:38 P.M. Call from Travis, cowboy from Colorado. I think I love him. Then wonder if it's because he's 1,500 miles away. Decide I'm a sicko.

5:45 P.M. Feeling a bit peckish. Go to grocery store. Notice two cute guys. Follow one to frozen foods, where other cute guy is waiting. Shall we have lima beans tonight? first guy asks second guy. Second guy bursts into tears. You know I hate lima beans, he says.

6:04 P.M. Three messages on machine. Mother, Rita, Chris. Call mother back. She's sad, doesn't have boyfriend. All the men like younger women, she says, you must have a million guys. I laugh mirthlessly.

6:52 P.M. Call Chris. Husband having affair, he admits all.

7:45 P.M. Hang up. Read magazine article "How to Spot a Heartbreaker." Take notes.

8:15 P.M. Call Rita back. She's sad, doesn't have boyfriend. We decide to go dancing later.

8:30 P.M. Greta calls. She has made decision to call cute guy from last night.

9:23 P.M. Cleo calls. Date over already. Seems guy suddenly had massive anxiety attack, complete with vomiting and hyperventilating, then admitted he was already living with someone. And ran out door. Cleo wonders if I have any Valium. I'm all out.

9:40 P.M. Amanda calls. Has decided to stop seeing self-centered wimp.

9:50 P.M. Chris arrives, in tears.

10:01 P.M. Greta calls. She called cute guy. He couldn't place her. She's depressed. Wonders if she should see shrink.

10:22 P.M. Chris's husband arrives. They fight. I retreat to bathroom.

10:35 P.M. Rita arrives, joins me. Terrific sound of breaking glass from living room. We cower in bathroom.

10:58 P.M. Chris and husband leave after deciding on marriage counseling. I sweep up.

11:10 P.M. Amanda calls. Has decided self-centered wimp is better than nothing.

11:45 P.M. Rita and I go to local honky-tonk.

1:30 A.M. Lead singer in band dedicates song to me. I wonder how he knows my name and grow concerned.

2:30 A.M. Lead singer dedicates another song to me. I'm becoming fascinated.

3:05 A.M. Rita, drunk, decides to go visit ex-boyfriend. She disappears into night.

4:20 A.M. Arrive home, singer in tow. Also road manager. We three sit in my living room, chat. I wonder what the hell.

5:00 A.M. Road manager pulls me aside for confidential word. Lead singer has wife waiting back at hotel, he says.

5:02 A.M. Lead singer and road manager leave, awakening landlady.

6:00 A.M. Go to sleep. Have dream.

DREAM

Lenny stared around the locker room morosely. Everything was as it should be, but a familiar ache had started in his groin and wouldn't let up. How much longer? he wondered to himself. How long can a red-blooded male put up with this shit? Frank came in, whistling and bouncing a basketball. Lenny perked up.

"Hey, Frank, heard anything about us going aboveground? I'm going bananas."

"Hey, Lenny my man, I keep telling you. Patience, my man."

"But hey, Frank, we've been down here so long, the broads up there must be ready for us by now. If they ache inside half as much as I do . . ."

"Is Lenny bitching again?" Larry yelled, his attention momentarily diverted from a huge Advent screen.

"Look at him," Lenny said contemptuously, "eating peanuts, chugging beer, watching an old tape of Super Bowl '79. Happier than a pig in shit."

"Fucking right," said Larry, belching contentedly.

"Well, I'm tired!" Lenny shouted, pounding his fist on his locker, which sported several photos of Loni Anderson. "I mean, I know it made a lot of sense for us to go underground. Those dames up there had got real weird and uppity after women's lib. I know that. I know how when Big John first discovered these huge unused caverns under the city it seemed like a helluva good idea for us all to gradually disappear, to bring those broads to their knees. But shit, man, it's been *years!* They must be ready for us by now. They must be *drooling*, man!"

"Hey, man," said Frank soothingly, "doesn't Big John, our esteemed leader, know what he's doing? Hasn't he kept us comfortable? Don't we have everything a man could desire? Hell, man, we can watch football, basketball, baseball, even *hockey*, twenty-four hours a day! In peace! We have unlimited peanuts and kegs of brew! We got locker rooms and after-shave! Plenty of jockstraps! Smelly cigars! We got softball teams! We got Merle Haggard records! What don't we got?"

"Pussy," said Lenny hollowly.

"Aw, Lenny, man," said Larry, tearing his eyes away from a spectacular run by Lynn Swann, "try and remember what it was like up there. Remember how we couldn't score unless we pretended to be all sensitive and wimpy? How we had to learn to cook fettuccine Alfredo? How we weren't allowed to say broad or chick? How we had to love 'em for their *minds*? How they'd sock us in the jaw if we didn't give good head?"

"Hey, guys, you know what I heard?" piped up Carl, who had just emerged from the showers after a rousing game of Ping-Pong. "I heard they're starting to claw each other's eyes out over us again. Oh, yeah, the chicks are going mental. I hear that every time you turn around there's a newspaper article called 'Where Are All the Men?' or 'A Good Man Is Hard to Find and Why.'"

"A hard man is good to find," smirked Frank.

Carl grinned and snapped his towel playfully at Frank. "I even heard that Morgan—remember Morgan, that fat awful guy with lousy breath who we sent surface-side on a groundhog mission last week?—well, I heard that a model, an actress, and a mud wrestler were killing each other over him. I heard that the model got down on her hands and knees and *begged* Morgan to go home with her."

"Holy shit," said Frank, his eyes glazing, "a model on her goddamned knees. Holy shit."

"I feel like I'm turning into one of those albino alligators down here," Lenny said, staring at his pasty-white hands.

"Big John says just a few more months, Lenny," said Carl, "and the broads will be under control."

"No they won't!" shouted Lenny, his eyes flashing. "We're never gonna get them where we want them! And I don't care anymore! I'll take what I can get." With a sudden spurt, Lenny went running toward the light.

It took six strong men to restrain him.

We thought we had them there, back in, say, 1971.

"We are women!" we screamed. "You can't fuck us over anymore! We don't *feel* like picking up your socks! We are *bored to death* listening to football stats! We only *pretended* we liked to go fishing! We don't *want* to smile inanely anymore! Ditto washing the floors and diapering! Ditto getting laid when we don't want to! Ditto batting our eyelashes!"

Pretty good stuff, we thought to ourselves, that ought to stop the bastards in their tracks.

And it did. Men are not stupid, or at least not too stupid to realize that if they didn't get sensitive *real fast*, they weren't going to get laid anymore. After all, we had put it rather neatly and succinctly: No equal pay, no pussy.

Men really got kind of cute. "*Mea culpa,*" they said to us as they assiduously mopped the kitchen floor and basted the pork chops. "We know we did wrong, but we didn't mean it. We know better now. We'll give you your space. We *know* where you're coming from."

But things, as they will, went sour. Men, used to quite a few years of power, found out that they weren't all that crazy about being penitent. Oh, it was a lark for a while, but all that washing up! All that giving up of jobs! All that foreplay!

What started as a barely discernible rumble became a deafening roar. "Fuck it!" men cried in unison all over the world, "we're not going to take this shit anymore!"

It was a devastating blow. One moment guys were running around not opening doors for us, the next minute they were either gay, psycho, or gone. The great boyfriend crunch had begun.

NO SEX, NO SANITY

We seem to be driving ourselves mentally ill over the boyfriend subject.

Here's how it happens: You, a girl, have the normal urges and desires. You want a man around—you want him to hold you, fondle you, soothe your troubled brow after a long day's work.

Yet somehow, there is no boyfriend in sight. You grow discouraged. The days pass, your needs are not met. You start kicking cans on the street and glaring at innocent fruit vendors. Your urges and desires are still there, throbbing and seething beneath the surface.

Throbbing and seething urges, when not released, give even the most stalwart and healthy girl morbid thoughts. She dwells. She smokes too many cigarettes. She rails against her fate. She begins to think that there must be something wrong with her.

As her depression continues, she becomes irretrievably positive that there *is* something drastically wrong with her, and she calls the men in the white coats to take her away.

"If only I were a little prettier," she says to the men in the white coats, "and had better skin, and weren't a seething mass of psycho-neurotic schizophrenic paranoic manic depressiveness, someone would probably love me."

Wrong! Very wrong!

Having a boyfriend is no proof of
(a) sanity
(b) desirability.
Ugly women have boyfriends, mean women have boyfriends, hopelessly insecure women have boyfriends, stupid women have boyfriends, women covered with hideous warts have boyfriends.

We cannot, as much as I think it is right and just that we should, have our cakes and eat them too. We cannot be the independent women that feminism has helped us realize we want to be and still judge ourselves in terms of whether or not we happen to have a man around the house. Boyfriends can no longer be
(a) status symbols
(b) indispensable
(c) meal tickets.
(Especially meal tickets. I've known otherwise sensible girls to pass up perfectly reasonable fellows just because this perfectly reasonable fellow didn't make as much money as she did. This is not fair.)

The State of the Male Psyche

What with all these sex-role upheavals, men are a mess. They've been taught all their lives to act one way, and suddenly they're told they must act completely differently. They are strung out. Angry. Scared.

"Men," says my friend David, who should know, "have no perceptive power, no intuition, and no control. How can we help acting stupid?"

Of course, men could have these things if they wanted. But they don't know what they want, except they're pretty sure they want to run away.

This leaves all of us in a pretty pickle. Men scared, women angry. Women scared, men angry. We don't know what to say to each other anymore, even talking about the weather can be a bit fraught:
He: Nice day, although it's looking a bit cloudy over to the west.

She: What are you trying to do? Patronize me or what? You think I can't see those clouds? I don't need *you* to point them out to me.

Or

SHE: I really hope we have good weather this weekend.

HE: Look, if this is your way of leading up to something, forget it. I already have plans for this weekend, and the last thing I need right now is a commitment.

SOLUTION?

We'll just have to wait for the dust to settle.

But even now, a light is flickering at the end of the tunnel. The strongest, smartest, and bravest men are coming around at last. They are putting their fears behind them and striking devastating blows against wimpdom by admitting that, in fact, we are all in this together. It takes fortitude to do this, and we must encourage them.

All we have to do is hang in there.

Unless, of course, we feel like giving up and turning into sweet, subservient yes-girls again.

3

How to Find Someone to Fall in Love With

Just be yourself.

—YOUR MOTHER

There are certain magazines which should be avoided. They call themselves "women's" magazines, which is absurd, since their complete *raison d'être* is the care and feeding of the male. How to make him happy in bed, how to choose his socks, how to tell if he's screwing his secretary and how to prepare his income tax returns are, according to these magazines, topics deemed monumental in importance.

Yet even I, when in the throes of an exasperating love affair, have been known to rush to the newsstand and mainline articles like "How to Tell if He *Likes* Your Breasts—A Leading Psychiatrist Explains All!"

The results of this madcap behavior are invariably disheartening.

I shall never forget the time when, fresh from the avid consumption of "How to Turn Him On over the Telephone—A Noted Courtesan Tells All!" I called Rex, a noted he-man, at his office.

"Hello, darling," I said when he answered, "I want to trace feathery kisses down your spine."

"Oh, hi," he said, "listen, I'm in a meeting, can I—?"

"I throb for you," I continued, as the particularly trenchant article said I should. "I ache all over. I want you to take me right now, even as we speak."

"This is a joke, right? Could you hurry up with the punch line? I've got a roomful of—"

"Just the thought of you turns me into a mass of lust."

"And it was nice talking to you too, Herb, give my love to the wife and kids," he said and hung up.

I stared at the phone receiver in dismay. This wasn't what was supposed to happen. According to the Noted Courtesan, Rex was supposed to stop whatever triviality he was doing and rush right to my bedside with roses and champagne.

Cleo recently told me that she spent four years not brushing her teeth in the proximity of a man because a certain article in a magazine told her men hated to see a woman swirl water around in her mouth.

And Rita still remembers, with significant horror, how she once simpered to a man at a cocktail party, "I'll give you the olive in my martini if you'll give me a match," because a magazine told her to.

Not only is it degrading to follow the advice of noted courtesans and psychiatrists—it doesn't work. All men are not the same. All women are not the same. So why do we blindly follow any inane advice which wafts our way? Why are you reading this book? Why am I writing it?

Because we're so achingly impressionable. We'll go to any lengths to make ourselves palatable. We ignore the still, small voice of our famous intuition. We have no faith in ourselves. I have never met a woman who, deep down in her core, really believes she has great legs. And if she suspects that she *might* have great legs, then she's convinced she has a shrill voice and no neck. Not one woman over seventeen has any faith in her skin tone, and no woman over thirty can ever regard her upper arms with equanimity.

Test this for yourself. Walk up to any woman on the street and say, "You know something, sweetheart? You'd look an awful lot better if you lost fifteen pounds. And do you really think that hair style is becoming? Don't you know *anything* about bone structure?

Anyway, with ankles like yours, I wouldn't bother to leave the house."

Instead of the proper response, which would be to deck you, nine out of ten women will apologize, burst into tears, and run away.

We're all hideous, that's what we are, and it's truly gratifying that anyone at all ever wants to go to bed with us. So we search like ferrets for the *key*, for that special knowledge that will make us appear to be the femme fatale we dream of being. We buy magazines that tell us how to act and what to think. We read advice columns that tell us what to do. We go to the movies and study Diane Keaton's mannerisms. We try to develop interesting personality traits. But not *too* interesting—we wouldn't want to intimidate.

Yet somehow, we're never good enough. Horrible lumps is what we are. Colorless blobs. Frowsy frumps.

This is what is known as a bad attitude. The kind of attitude that leads us to try to be someone else.

If you try to be someone else long enough, you forget who you are. You forget that you're the one who likes clams casino and Monty Python. You're not sure if you like blue or not. If someone asks you if you'd like a cup of coffee, you don't know. The color of your eyes escapes you.

The cause of this severe confusion is obvious when one stops to think about it:

FAULTY UPBRINGING

When Everygirl was a little girl, she learned a valuable lesson: She couldn't get what she wanted by asking for it. Being a good little Everygirl meant shutting up and pleasing others.

"But Johnny hit *his* friend over the head with a baseball bat and you didn't lock *him* in the attic for three months," Everygirl complained to her mom.

"But Johnny is a *boy*, dear," Mom explained. "Johnny gets to do stuff like that because when he grows up to be a man he will have to be strong and brave and hit other men over the head with a baseball bat when they try to steal his TV set."

"What'll I do when someone tries to steal *my* TV set?" Everygirl wondered.

"You'll get your man to hit him over the head with a baseball bat," Mom answered promptly.

Don't blame poor Mom, she's paid to say that, she doesn't really want to.

By the time Everygirl is pubescent, she has it figured. All her efforts at straightforwardness have been met with stony indifference, whereas all her little cutenesses and wheedling have netted her new shoes, a clock radio, and a lavender prom dress. She's learned to become an ace manipulator, our Everygirl. She's studied those in power and figured out how to get them to like her. She's learned how to sneeze like a kitten and blush prettily when confronted with a carburetor.

Eventually Mom feels compelled to come across with the goods.

"Just be yourself," Mom whispers furtively to Everygirl on the evening of Everygirl's first date with an actual college boy, when Everygirl is so frazzled she makes eight trips to the bathroom in four minutes and absently peels off all her nail polish.

"Just be yourself, Everygirl," Mom will whisper again. She's trying to tell her something of utmost importance. But it's too late.

"Oh, *Mom!*" Everygirl will whine, "how can I be myself? Who am I?" Poor Everygirl hasn't a clue. Her true nature has been plowed under by too many smiles, pretty murmurings, gentle pleadings, self-deprecating giggles.

This is a hell of a note.

The irony here is that to find someone to fall in love with, you have to know who you are.

Don't say "That's easy, I'm the one with the lousy nose and chubby legs who can't sing a note," since that describes all of us except Tina Turner. You have to embark on an all-out study.

START SIMPLE

Ask yourself the following questions:
Do I prefer Martha's Vineyard to Las Vegas?
Would I buy an herbal tea?
Would I ever consider setting my hair?
Do I regard Picasso as a fabulous artist?
Would you ever catch me at an EST meeting?
What are my thoughts on emerald brooches?

Do I prefer Miles Davis to Mick Jagger?

Do I jog?

Don't cheat. Don't think to yourself "Harry simply loves Miles Davis, and I love Harry, so I love Miles Davis too." We are not concerned with Harry's thoughts at the moment.

Eventually, if you apply yourself rigorously to the task, you'll get down to the basics. You'll find out if you prefer Wodehouse to Woody Allen, if you like watching television more than climbing mountains, if you want children, if you even want a relationship.

Make sure you go about all this with affection, or you'll blow the whole thing. Think of yourself as a terrifically engrossing mystery novel.

The difference in your personality will be startling and gratifying. Now that you know that you prefer *marrons glacés* to floating island, you'll start regarding yourself as a pretty damned fascinating human being. There will be a new, jaunty spring to your step. You'll pick up *Cosmopolitan* one day and wonder what you could ever have seen in it. Your eye will fall casually on an article entitled "How to Tap His Secret Appetites—A Noted Cook Reveals All!" and a small smirk will cross your lips as you throw the magazine down with gentle contempt. Hidden appetites indeed! Who are they kidding? Not you, that's for sure.

Pretty soon the whole world will get the benefit of the New You. You'll start sending back overdone steaks with a few choice syllables to any supercilious waiter who dares to raise an eyebrow. You'll tell surly telephone operators where to get off. The man at the hardware store will think long and hard before shortchanging *you*.

It's even possible that when your hairdresser decides to turn you into a low-rent version of Dolly Parton, you'll simply throw a hairbrush at him, instead of smiling wanly and handing over half your inheritance. (This may be too much to hope for.)

You'll also notice a marked change in the attitudes of your friends. Some will be pleased, others irritated.

"What's got into you?" the irritable ones will ask. "You always used to be so easy to please, so willing to sit around and listen to our problems. Now you always want to go dancing until dawn with wild Texans. Don't you care about us?"

"Well," you'll say, "I'm just learning to have a good time, is all."

"Don't bother," they'll say. "It's depressing, you running around singing all the time. Also, whatever could have possessed you to wear bright-yellow high heels?"

(This stuff really happens. I had a dear friend once, let's call her Susan. Whenever Susan and I met for lunch, she'd say, in a voice rife with sympathy, "What is it? You look so *depressed*." Even if I was feeling fine, I'd always be convinced Susan had discerned an untapped vein of misery, and that I really was, unbeknown to myself, deeply despondent. Susan would listen to my laments happily for hours. Then, one fine day, I phoned her to tell her all sorts of wonderful things that had been happening to me. She accused me, in no uncertain terms, of chewing her ear off. After about seven minutes. It occurred to me that with friends like her, who needs mothers?)

Prune these alleged friends ruthlessly from your life. You need all the positive reinforcement you can get. You need friends who think you're fabulous, an angel in human shape, and a breath of springtime.

As this new self of yours starts burgeoning, you'll find out, to your amusement, that you're not really so desperate to find someone to fall in love with after all. You won't, in fact, be a hollow shell, just waiting for someone to come along and fill you up, someone to make you whole. You won't be needy.

Neediness does tend to put your average male off, and he's right. A needy person is a difficult person, a manipulative person, a self-absorbed person. We've all known needy men, and we've always shunned them. Usually a girl who is needy does not even notice that the man next to her may have a few problems of his own and will take all sorts of things personally. Witness the following conversation:

NEEDY PERSON: What time will you be over tonight?

MAN IN QUESTION: That's what I'm calling about. I have a presentation to make tomorrow morning and I'm as nervous as a cat on hot bricks. I think I should stay home and work. How about tomorrow?

N.P.: Oh, God. I was really looking forward to this. I just don't know what to say.

M.I.Q.: How about "Okay Harvey, tomorrow will be just ducky."

N.P.: Maybe I could come over and cook for you and massage your neck when you get tense.
M.I.Q.: It wouldn't be worth it. I'm in a terrible mood. I'll snap your head off.
N.P.: Don't you like having me around?
M.I.Q.: Jesus Christ.
N.P.: Oh, I see. You've got another girl coming over tonight and you're afraid to tell me.
M.I.Q.: I resent that, I really do. Didn't we just spend the last three nights together?
N.P.: Terrific. I guess now you're saying you're spending too much time with me. You want to cut it down. You need your freedom. You need your own space.
M.I.Q.: Why do I suddenly feel as if I'm in a Joan Crawford movie?

Nobody wants to be in a Joan Crawford movie. Anybody who's anybody wants either to be Cary and Rosalind in *His Girl Friday* or Bill and Myrna in *The Thin Man*. Or even Dudley and Liza in *Arthur*, or Burt and Sally in *Smokey and the Bandit*. Joan Crawford movies are riddled with tearstained pillows and broken promises and no fun at all. Better even to be in a Neil Simon comedy, then at least you get a few snappy comebacks.

But I digress.

Here's the worst thing of all about a needy person: She (or he) hands over all the power to her (or his) love object without so much as a whimper. It may be true that everyone loves power, but not many want it handed to them on a silver platter. Where's the fun in that?

Another thing: You know how people are always saying that nobody will love you until you love yourself? Presbyterian ministers say it all the time. Well, it's not true. Utter rubbish, in fact. Even if you totally despise yourself, you can always scratch up a few suckers who will love every hair on your unworthy head.

But you'll hate them for it. If you think of yourself as a loathsome excrescence, the only man who will satisfy you is one who treats you accordingly.

We come, alas, to another personal anecdote.

Once, immediately after I had broken up with a sadistic menace named Brian (he used to leave other women's panties lurking in his bathroom, and lipstick-stained cigarettes—not my color—in the ashtray next to his bed), my self-confidence was shattered to bits, and I met Jake.

Jake was a big, burly angel, funnier than George Burns, cuter than Waylon Jennings, sweeter than a milkshake. He had a drawl like dark, hot honey. And he loved me. Thought I was the greatest. He showered me with roses, sent me impassioned postcards, and always knew when I needed a hug.

At first, I liked Jake fine. He amused me and made me forget about Brian's atrocities. Although things seemed a bit too easy without any *Sturm und Drang* business. We found the same things funny, and he never even minded that I was addicted to going to all-nite supermarkets at 4 A.M.

Pretty soon I started thinking that Jake must be a ninny. He liked me, didn't he? And I was an utter pimple, wasn't I?

It got worse. Pretty soon the poor man couldn't do a thing right. His crooked smile bothered me. Why couldn't he smile straight like other guys? The way his beard curled became vaguely distasteful to me. His shirts, I felt, showed a lack of subtlety.

The more he loved me, the more disdainful I got. Finally I fled from him completely. What a fool I was! When self-hatred strikes, it cripples fine minds and fit bodies. Jaunty girls turn to cowering jelly.

Now nobody's saying that you shouldn't be insecure. *Everybody in the world is insecure, not only you.* Even Jackie Onassis must wake up some mornings and burst into tears when she looks in the mirror. To be insecure is to be human.

But insecure is the worst you should be. On a bad day, be insecure and worry about the curve of your eyebrows. On a good day, know for a fact that you're the most scintillating human in the world. And before you know it, the man of your dreams will come moseying into your life, nice as you please.

At which point you must remember to flirt with him.

How to Flirt

It must be said, and now is a good time, that no matter how captivating a woman is, men do not usually fall, as if from trees, into her lap while she's sitting around her apartment. Especially now, during these lean years, one must flirt. Passivity may have its virtues, but when you're looking for romance, you have at least to get out of bed.

Flirting is a zestful, invigorating pastime. It is the mental equivalent of doing twenty pushups and jogging five miles, since a good flirt must use her brain at about three times normal speed.

Like riding a bicycle or performing brain surgery, flirting is an acquired skill that, once you get the hang of it, is a piece of cake.

The first thing a successful flirt does is get it firmly fixed in her mind that she is God's gift to men. A cool self-confidence is not only attractive, it also saves a lot of effort—you don't have to waste a lot of valuable thinking time wondering whether you're good enough to be talking to such a dreamboat, and can instead actually listen to what the dreamboat has to say.

Then you must simply charm him from the trees by letting him know that you, and you alone, know that he is the most intriguing man on earth.

Say, for example, you're at your typical cocktail party and a vision in a black fedora swims into your ken. Do not parade up to him and say "Wanna get high?" Do not try to fell him with a flying tackle and drag him home. Do not propose marriage.

Use subtlety, the essence of charm. Watch him covertly for a while, giving him fleeting come-hither glances at regular intervals. (A come-hither glance is easy—it's just still and steady eye contact for a second or two longer than is proper.)

Then go and stand next to him just a little bit closer than you think you should. And be silent just a bit longer than you think you should. He will become intensely aware of you and slightly nervous. This is where you say something casually intimate, as if you've known him for years. Something along the lines of "Do you think that man in the green suit is wearing a corset?" Or "Is that a pistol in your pocket or are you just glad to see me?" No, perhaps not. You have to give him room for a snappy comeback. How about "This is the first time I've worn this dress, and I'm still not sure I like the bow-on-the-shoulder effect. What are your thoughts?"

Then he'll say something, then you'll say something, then there you'll be, making a date for the movies next Thursday.

Do's and Don'ts, Flirtingwise

—Never try to establish a successful flirtation when your hair is a mess.

—Tell jokes. Sparkling, witty, we're-in-this-together-and-nobody-else-knows-how-funny-everything-is kinds of jokes. If you can establish a co-conspiratorial ambiance, you're on to something good. If you can't, if he looks at you as if you're a Martian, you don't want him anyway.

—Do not brag. If you brag, you may as well be wearing a sandwich board that says, "I am massively insecure." Instead, be somewhat reticent, nay, mysterious, about yourself. No, do not even drop hints about your latest Nobel Prize, or how you just negotiated the movie deal of the century, or how you've just bought your own twelve-room condo. And never, ever, talk about how good you are in bed.

—Avoid clichés. Do not, for example, say, "How's the weather up there?" to a tall guy. I knew a girl who did that, and, for this particular giant, she was the final straw. He looked pained, said, "It's raining," and spit on her.

—Exude a cool but promising skepticism. You don't want to fall all over a fellow, but you do want him to realize that if he amuses you enough, he's in for a mighty good time. Try not to touch him more than fleetingly.

—If you notice something good about him, mention it. As Oscar Wilde once noted: "Women are never disarmed by compliments. Men always are. That is the difference between the sexes." But never lie. Don't tell a fellow his pectorals make you weak when all he has is a potbelly.

—Within reason, you may tease. But when you say, "Tell me, whatever possessed you to wear that sweater?" smile.

—Go with your instincts. The prime destroyer of flirtation is a morbid superconsciousness that edits everything one says. Be brave and say what you think, even something like "Well, we seem to be getting on splendidly so far, even if you *are* a Scorpio."

—If you feel tongue-tied, don't say anything. Opt for a compelling silence.

—If he's shy, ask him about point spreads. Point spreads, you may have heard, have to do with football games and such. I have never met a man, even a die-hard homosexual who refuses to believe in Mickey Mantle, who doesn't have his own point-spread theories. And I have never met a woman who understands them at all. It's obviously a secondary sex characteristic. He'll be happy to explain the whole thing to you for hours.

—Do not be afraid. Where will fear get you? Nowhere. What do you have to lose by trying to captivate the most devastating man in the room? Nothing. Will you die if someone rejects you?

—Don't worry about whether or not he's gay. Gay men enjoy talking to women, and will tell you if you have a piece of pimento stuck in your teeth. He'll let you know his persuasion soon enough.

WHERE TO FLIRT

The best place for a beginner to learn to flirt is in Texas. Not only is the sky there awe-inspiring, but you'll like Texans. Unlike most urban men, who get all perspiring and edgy when confronted with one of those newfangled "career" women who are successful and autonomous and adventuresome, the cowboy hitches up his belt, takes a swig of his beer, and stares at this new breed of woman.

She, of course, is regarding him nervously, wondering if she should have confessed to owning her own advertising agency and also to being a fairly well respected nuclear physicist.

"Well, how about that," the cowboy will say with his inevitable drawl. "I sure am impressed. I am awestruck. You are a real interestin' woman. Now come here."

It's very heartening.

Rita tells the tale of the man at the U-Totem in Austin, Texas, who sidled up to her and asked, "Darling, didn't I meet you on a hot and dusty night in San Antone?" She was a bit dismayed when she learned later that Mick Jagger said it first.

If you can't get to Texas, a nice Country-and-Western honkytonk will have to do. There's something about the soft strains of the pedal steel that brings out the silvery tongue in everyone. And when the band sings

I miss you darlin more and more every day
As heavens miss the stars above

With every heartbeat I still think of you
And remember our faded love . . .

everyone in the audience gets all goopy and weepy and the next
thing you know a fellow in faded jeans will be telling you that the
way your hair shines reminds him of the sun setting over the
Rockies.

The worst place to try flirting is in New York City. The men there
are a mite arrogant, since the women outnumber them by about
three hundred to one (a serious point spread). This makes every
New York Man, even a pear-shaped, churlish bore, think he's everybody. Men in New York are never yearning, never hungry. They all
have that sleek, well-fed look of a tiger who's already had his supper.
This can be daunting, and sometimes actually damaging, since the
only way to get your average New York man interested is to pretend
to hate him, which will get you nowhere at all in other parts of the
country, even Los Angeles.

Even worse than New York City is any singles bar anywhere.
People in singles bars are insecure people like you and me but, unlike you and me, they spend most of their waking hours pretending
they're not. They feel degraded going to these singles bars, and take
it out on everyone. A typical example of male repartee singles-bar
style is: "Lemme guess, you're a stew. Wanna show me your land-
ing pattern? Okay, you're a secretary, right? Take a letter. Take
me home."

Do not take *any* bar-flirting seriously. The man of your dreams is
not sitting morosely on a barstool in a darkened corner, downing
mescal and shouting to the piano player to play it again. The man
of your dreams has better things to do with himself. Possibly he's
negotiating a peace settlement in the Mideast, or snapping up
microchip futures, or catching the winning touchdown at the Super
Bowl.

So if you want to find this guy, simply get on with your life. He'll
appear. Oh yes he will. You always think he won't, that the rest of
your life is destined to be empty and bleak, and that pretty soon
you'll have to take up knitting and start wearing white lace caps,
but no. Suddenly he'll enter stage left, when he's good and ready.
And when the stars are good and ready. And when your friends are

good and ready to break your kneecaps if you don't stop moaning about being lonely.

He'll probably be the guy who smashes into you on the street corner when you're carrying three bags of groceries.

After the two of you have gathered up all the soup cans rolling down the street, don't forget to get his phone number.

4

Sex Tips #1–
Remedial Sex Tips

Some girls are, no kidding around, really sophisticated. Advanced fellatio, a subject still grappled with by the finest minds in the country, is mere child's play to them. They have more exotic problems—how to turn a broom closet into a dominatrix's den, or what to do when the object of their desires turns up in pantyhose.

But some of us are pretty naive. We still read the instructions inside the Tampax box just in case. In this chapter we'll cover the basics, nothing fancy, no frills.

How to Enjoy Sex

You just do, that's all. Something in your glands makes you want the stuff, and when you get it, you like it.

Unless, of course, you're blocked. You want to enjoy sex, you know you're supposed to, and you've got a strange inkling that you actually could if you sincerely tried. But there's something murky, something sordid in your mind that's preventing you from having the time of your life. Possibly something psychological.

The first thing to do in this situation is to put sex out of your mind completely. Pay no attention to it. It will not go away. Sex is a perverse little devil, and the minute you ignore it, it has a serious temper tantrum and tries every trick in the book to get you to notice. It clamors for your attention until it gets it, at which point it disappears. So don't even watch your sexual urges out of the corner of your eye. Feign indifference.

Say, for example, you happen to be sitting on your sofa, watching television with a swell guy.

Things are going along pretty well. A particularly scary moment of Mary Tyler Moore comes on, you get nervous and grab his wrist. He comforts you by putting his arm around you and nuzzling your neck. You like this neck-nuzzling business so much you bite him jauntily on the shoulder.

Next thing you know his hand is tracing his initials on your knee, at which point he realizes you're wearing silk stockings and decides to investigate further.

You like this fine, and give him kisses. Little, tentative nibbling kisses, pretty good stuff. Rhoda is telling Mary a particularly funny joke ("Why eat this candy bar? Why don't I just apply it directly to my hips?"), but you've lost interest, because suddenly your tongues are seriously intertwined. He puts his hand on your breast. . . .

And then you get nervous. You start having this ridiculously ornate and complex inner monologue.

Should I run to the bathroom now and put in my diaphragm?

What's he gonna do when he sees my lumpy knees?

Should I grab his crotch yet?

What if he hates my tits?

And there you are. Passion has ceased.

It's as if you have suddenly been split in two, and one of you is doing all sorts of great things on the sofa, while the other you is sitting there over in the corner, notebook in hand, critiquing the situation.

You'll never have a good time this way. But don't feel stupid about this, it happens to everybody. Diane Keaton had the same problem in *Annie Hall*. And if it can happen to Diane Keaton in a hit movie for which she won an Oscar, it's nothing to be ashamed of. You've just been letting sex get the upper hand. Letting it rule your life. So what if you have lumpy knees or strange tits? Some of the best girls do. These are problems you should give your attention to while filing your nails, not when there's a hot number on your sofa. So whistle a little tune to yourself, twiddle your mental thumbs, and show sex that you're not paying any attention. It will then attack you with renewed vigor.

Unless, of course, you suffer from chronic sexual guilt.

SEXUAL GUILT

Myriads of girls are plagued by this embarrassing syndrome. To find out if you are, take this quick quiz:

1. Grabbing a man's penis is
    (a) a decent way to start off an evening
    (b) nice work if you can get it
    (c) a terrific ice-breaker at a dull dinner party
    (d) disgusting and bad

2. If I wake up naked in bed with a man, I
    (a) grab his penis
    (b) jump out of bed, brush my teeth, then come back and grab his penis
    (c) rub up against him and demand breakfast
    (d) grab my clothes and run screaming from the room

If you answered (d) to either of the above, you are suffering from sexual guilt.

More often than not, sexual guilt is deep-seated. This means that, ever since you were a child, your mother has been implying (in all sorts of subtle and nefarious ways) that sex is disgusting, dirty, nasty, vile, reprehensible, shameful, and creepy. Mothers do this all the time. They can't help themselves, poor dears, it's an occupational hazard of being a mother. They figure if they didn't say this sort of stuff, you'd be cavorting with burly, tattooed ex-cons the moment their backs were turned, getting pregnant and moving to a tedious trailer park in Idaho.

The cure for sexual guilt is simple: Get over it. Unless your mother was a psychopath, or your Uncle Ernie seduced you when you were eleven, you probably won't need extensive therapy. You must just acknowledge deep in your heart of hearts that *people are supposed to fuck.* It is our main purpose in life, and all those other activities—playing the trumpet, vacuuming carpets, reading mystery novels, eating chocolate mousse—are just ways of passing the time until you can fuck again. Well, maybe not eating chocolate mousse. If it is made with good Swiss chocolate and topped off with Devon cream, eating chocolate mousse is almost as good as fucking. But I digress.

Why do you think your parents made you go to bed so early? The minute your innocent childlike lashes fluttered shut, Mom and Dad fell on each other with crazed, unbridled passion. They just didn't happen to mention it to you.

A footnote here: Do not attempt to get over sexual guilt by inviting every tattoo-laden, burly ex-con you see into your bedroom. Take things slowly. Don't go any further than feels comfortable. Hold hands with a guy until you are utterly convinced that holding hands is not depraved. There's no hurry. Eventually you'll be fucking with your basic unbridled passion, like you're supposed to.

FATHER FIXATION

You're probably father-fixated. Most girls are at one time or another. It's almost impossible to believe when you look at the guy with his bald pate and beige polyester leisure suit. But once Dad wore terrific sharkskin suits, so now, every time you see a great sharkskin suit, your mind gets all tangled and confused and strange, and you don't know what to do. That's a father fixation, another cause of sexual guilt.

"You seem to be reacting to your boyfriend as if he were your father," your shrink may say stonily (unless she is a strict Freudian, in which case she'll shut up and wait until you think of it yourself, a process that usually takes ten years. This is why strict Freudians have such lovely summer houses).

This is just another little thing you must get over. It's really a common problem, so common that it's boring. People tend to yawn when they hear about father fixations, and you don't want that, do you? Of course you don't. Nobody chooses to be tedious.

INFERIORITY COMPLEX

Feeling insecure is another surefire way of spoiling a good time. If you happen to notice yourself thinking, "What could that hunk possibly see in me? Is there something the matter with him? Is he the kind of hunk who likes to do charity work?" you may well be suffering from lack of self-esteem.

In which case you must go back and read Chapter Three with feeling. And don't tell me your dog ate it or a mugger stole it or you dropped it in a puddle on the way to school. Chapter Three is nestling, nice as you please, just a few pages back. This book is not *Lady Chatterley's Lover*, you can't just skip to the dirty parts.

Suffice it to say that if you feel an insistent erection pressing against your thigh, this guy is hot to trot. And you, being the human being within closest proximity, are the object of his desires. Get on with it.

But then again, you may not be suffering from any sort of guilt or weirdness at all.

BOREDOM

Sometimes the reason for lack of sexual interest is lack of interest. There you are, sitting on this couch with this great guy. You know he's great because your friend Cleo told you she'd give up a Pulitzer if only this guy would give her a tumble. Your actual sister has confided that this fellow turns her into a puddle of lust. So you figure you've got to be interested, right?

Don't talk yourself into anything. One girl's chocolate mousse is another girl's beef jerky. Maybe the guy has streaky butterscotch-colored hair, and you fancy crisp black curls.

Marta, for example, becomes almost uncontrollable when confronted with short, funny Jewish men with cute asses. If a man is over five feet five, she is left cold.

I once was involved with two (2) men. Both were pleasant, wealthy, and presentable. Don was thin, well-muscled, bearded, and made heart-rending chili. He would phone me every day and croon vile songs in my ear. One day it was "Feelings," the next it was "Send In the Clowns." He had an unerring penchant for total silliness, and I was crazy about him.

But I could not sleep with him. I kept trying to want to. We'd go out to dinner—he always knew about some unknown yet intriguing Cajun restaurant—and we'd become completely immersed in some exotic, far-reaching dialogue riddled with wit and empathy. And yet, as the evening drew to a close and it was time to go to his place or mine, I would invariably develop a sick headache. The chemistry was just not right.

Richard, on the other hand, was an arrogant social climber. He was the kind of fellow who was forever telling you how rich he was, how many famous people doted on him, how many limos he'd been in that week. Not only that, but he had the unpleasant habit of latching on to pet phrases. Anyone he didn't like he called a "dog's breakfast." He referred to Quaaludes as "disco biscuits." I ask you. He thought he was hilarious, and he put me to sleep.

"But," I hear you say, "he must have been great-looking, a regular Adonis." Hah.

He was red-faced and paunchy. His eyelashes were insipid. The man was a dog's breakfast.

And I couldn't get enough of him. He used to like to take me to places where it was rumored that Jackie O was about to appear, and I would sit there, deeply bored and consumed with lust.

Granted, I am a sicko. But that's not the point, which is that you never know what—or who—is going to turn you on, and it's no good trying to pretend you are when you aren't.

(I would like to say here, just to clear things up, that I am not solely interested in red-faced paunchy bores. I had a momentary lapse, is all.)

MASTURBATORY TECHNIQUES

A singularly effective method of transcending sexual guilt and confusion is to masturbate with great frequency. Masturbation is not only good for helping you understand your body's responses, it is also great fun.

You probably already know how to masturbate. Possibly you've been to masturbation encounter groups, an appalling concept. You may well be an Olympic-class masturbator by now.

Then again, maybe not. I myself, little Miss Sex Tips, knew nothing until I was twenty-four. I finally got my nerve up to ask a couple of friends to help me with the finer points. It was pretty good.

The first thing to do is lie down and get comfortable. Turn off the TV, radio and, if you're really serious, the telephone. Take off your pants, you need to be able to let your legs wiggle freely. Then find your clitoris with your hand. You can't miss the little darling— it's that button at the front of your vagina. If you can't find it, consult a reputable physician or a friendly plumber. Then start playing with yourself. Most girls prefer to use the index and middle finger. Just fiddle about lazily, no need to get really serious yet.

Let your mind wander, and pretty soon some kind of filthy fantasy will pop into your head.

Let's see. Something like . . . You've been invited to Dubuque to give a lecture on neurosurgery. There you are, sitting on the plane, minding your own business and studying your notes, when the stewardess taps you on the shoulder.

"The captain and cocaptain wonder if you'd like to tour the cockpit," she says to you, smiling pertly.

"Why me?" you ask, vaguely disgruntled.

"They've heard that you're a famous brain surgeon and would be just thrilled to meet you," she trills.

"Oh, all right," you mutter, standing up and adjusting your fetching pearl-gray linen suit.

You follow her to the cockpit, where the pilot, who happens to strongly resemble Nick Nolte on a good day, greets you with a hearty handshake.

His copilot, who bears a striking resemblance to Mean Joe Green, gives you a jaunty salute.

"You can leave now, stewardess," the pilot says, and she does.

The pilot thinks perhaps you'd like to learn how to fly a plane, and straps you into his seat.

"You see that little dial right over there?" he asks huskily.

"Which one?" you ask, since there are so many dials and you want to get it right.

"Mumph," he answers, and you suddenly realize that he is on his knees, running his hands up your thighs and putting his head under your skirt.

You, of course, are taken a trifle off guard. This is not exactly what you were expecting. In fact, you let him slip your panties off and begin toying with you lightly but determinedly with his tongue before you whisper, "Quit that or I'll call the cops."

"There are no cops up here," pipes up the copilot, another county heard from. He seems unduly interested in the proceedings.

The pilot looks at you with pleading, melting blue eyes. "I'll stop if you want me to," he says, "but gee whiz, I want you so bad."

Poor thing, your heart goes out to him. "Oh, all right," you growl impatiently, "but get on with it. I've got a lecture to formulate."

He forces your legs apart and gets on with it, groaning happily. Next thing you know, the copilot is clamoring for attention. . . .

I seem to have got carried away. My fingers literally flew across the page at that last bit. I'm feeling a little feverish and, if you can spare me for a moment, I'm going to lie down.

There. That's better. One interesting side effect of masturbation is that it puts you immediately to sleep. A better soporific cannot be found. So from now on, never mind the hot milk business.

Some girls prefer to lie on their stomachs with a pillow pressed between their legs. God knows how they manage it, but they swear they do.

I personally will have no truck with vibrators, but I may very well be wrong. Marta, for example, has had a long and profoundly meaningful relationship with hers, and says it's the only way to do it if you have long fingernails.

"You know," she said to me one day, "the kind of orgasm you get that's really incredible, the kind that makes you think you're totally in love?"

"Vaguely," I said.

"Well, I had one of those the other day. It was amazing. The only thing is, it was with my vibrator. It made me wonder what life is all about, having one of those orgasms all by myself."

Makes you think.

Do you happen to know about the shower massage? Don't even waste a second glance on the stationary type that attaches to the shower head and stays there. What you're interested in is one of those babies with a long cord that enables you to apply it with abandon to all parts of your body. Adjust it halfway between spray and slow massage and put it between your legs. Adjust the water to warm. Within microseconds you will experience a strange yet familiar tingling sensation which will quickly escalate into one full-fledged orgasm after another. In fact, knowing you, you may go completely off your head, so make sure you have one of those rubber bath mats or daisies or something, and maintain a firm toehold.

After years of scientific research, I have come up with the complete clinical description of what an orgasm feels like:

An orgasm feels like that first rush of morphine after it's injected into the vein.

An orgasm feels like that moment between diving off a cliff and arriving in a clear lake.

An orgasm feels like the taste of a terrific plum.

An orgasm feels like sliding safe into home plate.

An orgasm feels like playing a perfect guitar solo.

An orgasm feels like finding a stunning lynx coat at a church rummage sale.

An orgasm feels like the first time you rode your bike without training wheels and the time you got a new puppy, combined.

Some of them are better than others, but all of them are okay.

BIRTH CONTROL

Your modern girl is often pondering the perils of birth control. As well she should be, since each and every method sucks. Consider the following:

Condoms: First of all, men hate them. There they are with a nice erection, all ready to put it someplace cozy and warm, and instead they have to sheath it in some sort of slimy, rubbery thing. Erections, which are sensitive creatures, often wilt at the very idea. But even if they do not, even if the desired cozy warm place is achieved, there is still this awful thing between the erection and its objective. Don't think a man can't tell.

You'll hate them too. They tend to bunch up and, instead of pleasurable friction, you get some sort of strange awful lumpiness rubbing against you. And even if they don't bunch up (which they do), they feel like rubber. Even if they're made of lambskin, they feel like rubber. And think of the poor lamb. Think of the poor lamb's mother.

Another irritating thing about condoms is that they tend to get holes in them. Sperm simply adore holes in condoms. They swim easily through them, up the Fallopian tubes, and attach themselves to the ovum with dispatch.

So there you are, in the middle of the night and a torrid scene of passion. You bite your lip and say, "Darling, are you sure that condom doesn't have a hole in it?"

"What?" he asks testily. Men hate questions like this.

"I don't want any stray sperm sneaking up my Fallopian tubes," you murmur.

"Jesus fucking Christ," he says, switching on the light. Then you both search the vile little thing for holes, a tedious activity at best. During this process you're bound to have a small tiff about whether you *really* care or are just leading him on, which will escalate into a huge battle—you bringing up the time he got drunk and made a pass at Gloria, him mentioning how you've never in your life been on time for lunch. This will inevitably culminate in one of you sleeping on the couch, or possibly even storming out into the night, muttering at the stars. So forget condoms.

At first glance, birth-control pills seem like a great idea. You pop one in your mouth each morning and never get pregnant. What could be more adorable?

But don't take them. Just don't, that's all. Beside the fact that they may cause blood clots, strokes, heart attacks, cancer of the breast, cervix, vagina or liver (I'm reading the label as I type this), dismenorrhea, amenorrhea, infertility, nausea and vomiting, abdominal cramps and bloating, breakthrough bleeding and spotting, migraines, depression, allergic rashes, infertility, high blood pressure, enlarged and tender breasts, spotty darkening of the skin, weight gain or loss, stomachache, yeast infection, asthma, convulsive disorders, water retention, jaundice, frequent urination, dizziness, nervousness, hearing problems, loss of scalp hair, change in sex drive, hearing problems, nasal inflammation, gum disease, cataracts, inability to use contact lenses, tiredness, backache, vaginal infections, inflammation of the pancreas, liver or colon, chorea, burning or prickly sensation, rheumatoid arthritis, or death—besides all that, they simulate pregnancy, and the only reason you stop taking them for five days is so that you think you're getting a period, which is not an actual period at all, just a psychological sop.

Also, lots of girls who take the pill get hairs on their chins. Long, coarse, dark hairs that are singularly unattractive and stupid. You don't need this sort of thing, you have enough problems.

IUDs are okay until they go wrong. Well actually they start right off being horrible. It hurts like surgery, having them inserted. We're talking real pain here, and lots of blood for days. They say it's easier to put an IUD in after you've already had a child, but they're nuts, and the treatment of actual pain is a boring reason to become addicted to Percodan.

Plus they tell you to check the string each day to make sure the damned thing is firmly in place. Not one girl I know who has had an IUD has ever been able to feel the string after the first six weeks. Somehow, some way, they get hopelessly lost in there. The only good thing about the string business is that if someone catches you unaware when you happen to be in the throes of masturbation, you can laugh airily and say, "Just checking for the string, doncha know. Have a pecan." Of course, you don't actually need an IUD to pull off this ruse.

Many incidents have been reported of babies being born with Mama's IUD clutched firmly in their fat little fists.

And then there are those irritating massive uterine infections. Penny tells a particularly amusing story of the time when, sick as a Doberman, she went to see a gynecologist.

"Hmmm," said the gyno, scratching his beard (he was one of *those*), "looks to me like you have a pretty massive uterine infection, caused by the IUD. It'll have to come out. Trouble is, it's got upside down somehow. I can't remove it without operating. I'll give you lots of antibiotics instead."

The antibiotics gave Penny a yeast infection, and the uterine infection recurred. She eventually went to stay with her mother-in-law, a fine woman, who nursed her back to health with organic rhubarb. When Penny was almost cured, her ex-husband popped in from nowhere, wanting his mother to cure the arthritic spurs he got from scuba diving. A poignant reconciliation ensued. Penny and Steve promised to love each other always and never to stray again. They went off to Sausalito together and were blissfully happy for three months, when Steve decided that, after all, he *really* wanted to get into acting. The cosmos works in mysterious ways.

If you have your tubes tied, you will immediately be overcome with remorse and decide that you must have children. You will begin adoption proceedings immediately, and will wait seven years for a suitable infant. You will then be forever plagued with the suspicion that little Phoebe's real father was, in fact, Charles Manson.

I once decided to use foam and was pregnant within a week.

The rhythm method is always a possibility, but you have to be awfully fond of thermometers, and quite good at math.

ZEN AND THE ART OF DIAPHRAGM INSERTION

There's nothing for it but to get yourself a diaphragm.

God, do I hate my diaphragm. Sometimes I can whisk it in in seconds. Other times it gets stuck in there at a strange angle and won't unfold no matter what. You always get gooky spermicide all over everything unless you use that crochet hook of an inserter, which Mary swears by, but which only comes with certain types of diaphragms and is just something else to worry about anyway.

I have a long-lasting relationship with my diaphragm, but it is peppered with some terrific fights. Here's one now:

ME: Get in there, you little bastard.

IT: Why should I? Just so you can get your rocks off with that sap? I'll bet he wears nylon jockey shorts.

ME: I happen to know he wears completely normal pale-blue briefs. Rita told me all. And anyway, what's it to you?

IT: What's it to *me*? *I'm* the one who bears the brunt of it, that's all. Especially since you *will* persist in doing it standing up. All that pounding is playing havoc with my flexguard.

ME: *Please* behave. He probably thinks I *died* in here.

IT: Go fuck yourself.

Of course I always win. But by the time I emerge, sweaty and victorious, from the bathroom, the fellow has become deeply engrossed in a rerun of M*A*S*H.

So what's a girl to do?

A girl must practice Zen. Only when you have achieved a higher level of consciousness will you be able to truly realize the essential rightness of when, why, and how to insert the diaphragm.

The first thing an aspirant on the road to enlightenment must realize is that there is no you, there is no diaphragm, that you and the diaphragm melt into the oneness of life's broad river. Only then can you practice the artless art, the unmoved movement, the undanced dance of diaphragm insertion.

When in the act of insertion, one must not let oneself be plagued by petty impatience, by the frustrations of the slippery rim. One must instead, like the Samurai, think of the great emptiness, which will eventually lead to the wondrous unfoldment. In other words, relax. Everything works if you let it.

When determining the time to insert the diaphragm, one must let the force flow through one and realize that there is no difference between sexual frustration and sexual fulfillment, between rejection and acceptance. "It" inserts the diaphragm, "it" decides whether or not one is to have sex.

One must not wonder, "Will we do it or not?" One must prepare oneself equally for both eventualities. If one inserts the diaphragm and then there is no sex, one must not feel disappointment. Conversely, one may have inserted the diaphragm and decide one doesn't feel like it after all.

To be a Zen adept, just insert the wondrous object whenever there is even a small possibility that one may have sex. After dinner is usually the optimum time. Otherwise one runs the risk of being in a continual state of unenlightened anxiety, asking oneself, "Should I run to the bathroom now?" after a prolonged kiss, and then, "How about now?" after one's blouse is unbuttoned.

Do oneself a favor. Put it in and forget it. You will or you won't get laid, but, like the Zen archer, you'll be ready.

5

Love and Other Phenomena

What is falling in love anyway? Is it when you wake up in the morning with His name resounding in your head? When you have to run to check your mascara six times in five minutes because He is about to ring your doorbell? Is it when somebody buys you an emerald brooch and you worry about whether he can afford it? Is it when you have an orgasm whenever he touches your nipple, when you usually need thirty-five minutes of serious cunnilingus? Is it when you feel kind of safe and warm and runny when he's around and cold and dry and nervous when he isn't? Is it when he walks into a restaurant with another woman and you think, "That must be his sister"? Is it when he walks into a restaurant with another woman and you think, "I'll put his eyes out with an icepick"? Is it when you start hugging total strangers on the street just because it feels right?

I was pondering just such questions when I visited Marta, a terribly sophisticated fashion designer with a heart of gold and a past that would make Liz Taylor green. She has put this past behind her and married a handsome, kindhearted comedian, but she still knows what she's talking about when she talks about love.

"He treats me like a dog," I complained to her, "and not even a respectable dog like a Saint Bernard. He treats me like a miniature schnauzer. But whenever I see him, my insides go all funny."

Marta put down her scissors and regarded me sympathetically. "What you have to realize, and quick," she said, "is that love is not that nauseous feeling you get in your stomach."

"It isn't?" I asked, dumbfounded.

"Not on your life," she said definitely.

Well, that certainly changed the complexion of things. I was always under the impression that once you got that nauseous feeling, that was It. You know the one I mean: Every time you think about him, which is approximately 80 percent of the time, your stomach does eight belly-flops and twelve backflips and four chinups all at once. It's kind of a good feeling, it gives you a bouncy step—but it can also make you want to throw up. And it's a feeling that can turn bad and mean and relentless, like when he disappears for a decade (which, when you're in the throes, means about ten minutes).

"I feel a stunning change of consciousness coming on," I said.

"About time, too," Marta said.

So if it's not that nauseous feeling, what is love anyway?

After years of rigorous scientific experimentation, I have concluded that being in love is when you go all weak:

Like the first time you heard the Rolling Stones. Or when you read *The Catcher in the Rye,* or ate the perfect *chile relleno.*

Going all weak is experiencing something that's just so perfectly wonderful, so beautiful, so *right,* that you think you're going to burst.

Every once in a while a man comes along who makes you feel like this.

I married a man because he used to do this inane little dance, his feet like whirling dervishes, which made me go weak.

And I'll never forget the first time I met Jake, the man I loved and lost. He was standing in the corner at one of those misbegotten Hollywood parties, guarding the beer like a surly Doberman.

"Why not circulate?" I said to my future fate. "The beer can defend itself."

He kissed my hand. "Take me away from all this," he implored, "there's people here whose souls are composed of dry ice. If I weren't a big burly man, I'd burst into tears. Do something quick. Let's go to Montana. Let's go to Palm Springs. Let's go to my house and see if we can find any drugs."

As far as speeches go, this may not have been much. But it made me go weak. So weak I forgot that in an hour I was to meet Rita, my best friend and partner in crime. We were, Rita and I, going to see Merle Haggard, pretty exciting. And it clean went out of my head when this silly man threatened to burst into tears. I went off with him.

Rita understood. She is a Texan, and knows how these things sometimes happen. And not only is she a Texan, but she's about eight feet tall with bright red hair and earrings that fall down so long they hit her shoulders. She calls everybody darlin' and can tell a fool from a thousand paces.

"I am *so* sorry, Rita," I said. "There was something about him that made everything else go out of my head."

"Darlin'," Rita said, "you are in *serious* trouble. The last time everything went out of my head like that was when I met my third husband, who was my final husband and probably the true love of my life."

"He was so silly," I said, "he made me go weak."

"Oh my goodness," Rita said.

Sometimes it's not so dramatic. Sometimes you have no idea you're in love until you're sitting at home one day, painting your toenails and musing, "I've gotta tell Frankie about that stupid thing that happened to me at the grocery store this morning. Frankie's the only one in the world who will get it. And also I'd better ask him if he thinks I should be a redhead."

And then suddenly, out of nowhere, you realize you've been in love with good old Frankie since time immemorial, that nobody else will do, and that you can't live without him. (Don't neglect to tell Frankie about this.)

The thing is, you've gotta wait for it. Falling in love is something that will happen to you once, twice, maybe three times in your life. And you can't convince yourself you are in love when you aren't. When you are you'll know it. Everything will just seem right, and there you'll be. (Don't bother trying to make it happen. You can flirt and wiggle and bat your eyelashes all over cocktail parties whenever you want to, but you must not get dejected if there is no response.)

Here's another way of telling: You know how you love your sister, or your kid if you have one, or your best friend? Well, love, after all, is love, so it's basically the same thing. Within reason, of course. Unless you're very weird indeed, you will not be wanting to rip all your sister's clothes off and cover her with steamy kisses, which you'd better want to do to the man you're in love with, or you're not in love with him.

And do not, at your peril, overlook the sense-of-humor question. You can't be in love with someone who doesn't have a sense of humor. You just can't. Unless you don't have one either, and that's a situation too macabre even to contemplate.

A sense of humor isn't everything. It's only 90 percent of everything. And since, like snowflakes or fingerprints, every person's sense of humor is different, people invariably fall in love because their senses of humor are uncannily similar. Both of them fall on the floor when the wine steward pronounces the Pouilly-Fuissé "audacious," and both are left cold by Charlie Chaplin movies. So if you laugh uproariously when confronted with tofu fritters, and your inamorato doesn't get the joke, you're on very shaky ground.

Even sex isn't as important. Oh, okay, yes it is. But anybody you're in love with is automatically a good lay. Even if he's objectively terrible, you can't get enough of him. (Well, not too terrible. Anyone who's really terrible in bed is suffering from advanced repression or is a junkie. If he's repressed, you can work on it. If he's a junkie, you're not in love, just self-destructive.)

More ways to tell if you're in love:

—If he dresses with an astonishing lack of style—bell-bottomed suede trousers with fringed vests, or polyester leisure suits with clip-on ties spring to mind—and you don't care. Not only don't you care, you actually let your friends see him. Not only do you let your friends see him, you let your *ex-boyfriend* see him.

—If you think his feet are cute.

—If one of your major fantasies about him involves shopping in supermarkets.

—If you know for sure that he's scared of spiders, anal-retentive about the cap on the toothpaste, can't swim, and faints at the sight of blood, and you love him just as much (but not more).

—If Nick Nolte calls you and says he can't live without you and you say, "Gee, Nick, I'd really like to see you and all, but I've met this fellow. Let me just tell you about his feet. . . ."

—If you feel smarter, prettier, funnier and happier when you're with him.

—If the idea of him being hurt fills you with dread and fury.

Depressed? None of the above stuff rings a bell? Being in love is not what you are, but you do know you feel *something*?

Be advised that there are other states of consciousness caused by men, none as transcendental as actual love, but what the hell, sometimes you're not ready for transcendence anyway.

Herein defined are other states of sexual arousal. Possibly you'll recognize one or more of them.

HORNINESS

The state of being horny (or randy, if you're English) is not always felt at its source, but can instead be manifested by blurry vision, mouth dryness, heart palpitations, prickling feelings in the knees, numbness in the extremities, the aforementioned nausea, or the ever-popular liquidity in the loins.

The following are the ten warning signs of horniness. If you check off more than one, you're riddled with it:

1. You exist.

2. When introduced to a man, any man, you immediately wonder what it would be like to take a shower with him.

3. When driving in a foreign sports car, you find yourself gazing contemplatively at the gearshift.

4. When going to the corner to buy a quart of milk, you change your outfit three times and carefully apply mascara, just in case.

5. You often ruminate on the possibility of setting a small fire in the living room, changing into a frilly negligee, and calling the fire department.

6. Merv Griffin begins to look good to you.

7. You frequent bars late at night even when you have early morning meetings to attend, and you drink beer with bourbon chasers even though you don't drink.

8. James Garner drives you into uncontrollable frenzies.

9. Instead of having breakfast, you masturbate.

10. You wonder if the twelve-year-old down the street is old enough yet.

There is no known cure for horniness, thank God, although getting laid provides a certain temporary relief. Rumor has it, however, that if you don't have sex for more than a year, something inside you atrophies and instead of wanting it you start raising Weimaraners instead.

INSTANT LUST

When you see someone across the room and suddenly know for a fact that he's the most wonderful man on earth, you've got instant lust on your hands. Something about the way his tie is knotted is infinitely intriguing to you, and the swell of his bicep causes inner turmoil. This is a happy but fleeting state of affairs. Usually your feelings die about thirty seconds after you get up the courage to ask him for the time, since almost invariably he can't speak English, and if he can, he always says, "Why, sure, little lady, it's eleven-thirty. Wanna get high?"

Don't bother thinking that instant lust will turn into the real thing. It may, but then you may also wake up one morning to find you're the Queen of Rumania.

A CRUSH

You had your first crush when you were twelve years old, right when you were first getting horny and had no idea what was happening. At that time, it was either your history teacher or Paul McCartney.

A crush is a passive love affair, without risk. They're great when you have a lot of work to do and have no time for reclining in someone's strong, capable arms, or having endearments whispered into your ear, or partaking in blissful sex. With a crush, you just fantasize instead. No muss, no fuss.

A crush can be delicious in its own anticipatory way, but one should also contemplate the possibility of getting up the nerve to make a pass at the crush-object. Otherwise you're just being lazy or too self-protective for your own good.

Often the crush-object has no idea of your intentions, which is why he saunters casually by the water cooler even though you're lurking there, making eyes at him. So be brave and ask him out to a movie.

INFATUATION

This is a tough one. When you're infatuated, you think you're in love but you're not. Your heart palpitates, you look into his eyes with great poignant mistiness, and you rip his clothes off at every available opportunity.

There is nothing wrong with this. Infatuation passes the time a lot better than the Movie of the Week, and it's a bit more real. But not that real. Seventy-seven percent of infatuation is based upon fantasy.

As long as the two of you are going for quiet walks along deserted beaches, or dancing the tango in Bahía, you're fine. But the minute one of you needs extensive root-canal work, forget it. Real life does not sit well with infatuation. Your beloved really doesn't want to know that you have a gas leak, and you, in your heart of hearts, couldn't care less if his agent hates his manuscript. In fact, if his agent does hate his manuscript, you're bound to go off him a bit, since he's not the Mr. Perfect those languid strolls in the sand led you to expect.

People who are experiencing infatuation are loath to admit it. "No, no, no, this is different," my buddy Cleo will insist after I point out that she has been in love seven times in one month. "Randy's *perfect*," she'll say dreamily.

Cleo is a good girl, a giant in the journalism field even though she stands five feet three. She has pale-blond hair, green eyes, a mean wit, and a strong penchant for romantic intrigue.

Three days later, Randy will turn out to be not Mr. Perfect at all, but a callow, insensitive weakling who cares more for his Honda than he does for Cleo. What she ever could have seen in him, she'll never know. But there's this other guy, Mike. A dream, an absolute dream. Which is absolutely the truth.

A good way of figuring out whether it's infatuation or love is to go away with him for the weekend. Make sure the weather report promises rain, sleet, or hail. Choose a place that's inaccessible by major highway.

By the time you've been lost for the third time and the windshield wiper has broken down, you'll be getting to know each other pretty well.

"Shouldn't we have turned down that funny little road we just passed?" you'll ask.

"Oh God," he'll moan, running his hands through those curls you once found appealing, "why didn't you tell me that a hundred yards back? You're supposed to be reading the map!"

"Well," you'll retort, "maybe *you'd* like to figure out these squiggly red lines!"

By the time you arrive at your destination, you'll be in fine fettle. Then, after three days of kicking around the hotel room, watching the raindrops splash gently against the beach cabanas, one of two things will happen:

You'll either both be reduced to monosyllabic, sullen grunts—grunts which, if they could speak, would be saying, "I must have been crazy ever to have thought your eyes were like limpid pools, you vile personage. Limpid pools, hah! Limpid sewers is more like it! What could I have been thinking?"—or, instead, you will have fashioned all the sheets and blankets into a makeshift teepee and be playing a particularly rousing game of Cowboys and Indians. In which case you're probably in love.

SERIOUS LIKE

You like him a lot. You're not in love, mind you, but he sure does brighten up the day. You like going to parties with him, he's a great Scrabble player, and you want to be with him every minute. But still, he is, you figure, not quite Mr. Right.

You may be correct. Maybe he's just a close approximation of Mr. Right, who will do very nicely until the real thing comes along.

But you may be wrong. You may be just scared of getting too close, scared of taking the risk, scared of getting hurt. Or maybe you think that falling in love makes the world turn into a rosy-pink cloud of cotton candy. This never happens. If it does, someone has slipped a strong hallucinogen into your orange juice.

Try giving the fellow a chance. A good way to start loving someone is to feel close to him. Let yourself go, what the hell. If it doesn't work out, you can always kill yourself.

OBSESSION

I don't have the heart to go too deeply into this right now. Rumor has it obsession will be touched upon heavily in a future chapter or two, since it is the number one killer of a good time and has reached epidemic proportions in girls all over the nation. Who knows? It might be a leitmotif throughout the book, and I believe it's the subject of the next chapter. Possibly the book should be called "Your Obsessional Desires: Fact or Fantasy or Both"? Or how about "Obsession and You: The Grisly Truth"? Or "I'm Okay, You're Obsessed"?

Actually, I'm obsessed, you're okay.

LUKEWARM LOVE

This state is not as tedious as it sounds. There are some men in this world who are wonderful but limited.

Maybe he's too young and looks at you blankly when you mention Jimi Hendrix. Maybe he's too old and never shuts up about Will Rogers. Possibly he lives in Nova Scotia and you don't like salmon. He could be married to someone else. He could have once been married to you.

Oh, you love him, you really do, only not enough to move to Nova Scotia and listen to Will Rogers stories.

This is fine. Nobody ever said it had to be all or nothing. And if they did, you weren't listening. Relationships like these can last happily for years, and are more satisfying and substantial than twenty torrid infatuations.

Make sure to keep in touch. There's nothing sadder than wondering, five years later, how old Fred is doing. Is he getting along well with his new wife? Do his kids have blond hair like his? Did he ever get to Thailand like he always wanted to? By the time you start pondering Thailand, you'll burst into tears of regret and nostalgia. Don't let this happen. Any kind of love at all is too precious.

HATRED

He's in love with you, you hate him. But you keep him around even though you think that if you have to look at his oily face one more time you'll puke. So why don't you get rid of him?

Because you're angry. You like to see men grovel. Crawl.

You tell yourself other things, like you'll just keep Harry around until someone better comes along. In the meantime, Harry washes your car, balances your checkbook, feeds your dog. He's a sicko himself, old Harry. Otherwise he wouldn't put up with this torture.

BOY-CRAZINESS

You're allowed to be boy-crazy until you're eighteen, or twenty-one if you were reared in a strict Methodist household. Teen boy-craziness is simply girlish high spirits.

When your young girl first discovers that boys are good for something besides writing in the snow and fixing her clock radio, she is at first surprised, then nervous, then pleased as punch. Short boys, tall boys, hairy boys, pimply boys, wimpy boys—she loves them all. She can't get enough of them. They fill her dreams.

But if you're thirty-two and still boy-crazy, we're talking arrested development (okay development, assume the position. You have the right to remain silent . . .). You're still thinking of boys every second. There's Bert, there's Roger, there's Larry. Your friends, even your shrink, get dizzy trying to keep track of the dramatis personae.

It's all because you were never a cheerleader in high school, and thus experienced the brain trauma that makes you think of all men as captains of the football team. In short, you still want to be popular.

Scratch any adult who suffers from boy-craziness and you'll find a woman who still sees herself as a pimply little person who could never keep her knee socks up. Men are collected like scalps just so she can prove her self-image wrong, and she still has the attention span of a fifteen-year-old.

If you have a sneaking suspicion that you're boy-crazy (some of the best of us have), the only thing you can do is get it through your head that you can never be prom queen. You're too damned old, for one thing. For another, pink tulle is not becoming. And that dreamy football captain is now balding and sells used cars.

This realization will make you sad at first. You'll fret and refuse to eat your granola. But, with a little time, you'll feel like a new woman.

When one is not precisely sure how to define one's romantic involvement, it is always useful to take the telephone test. Simply monitor yourself while talking to your best friend, making sure to note her responses. Then check your conversation against the samples below and you'll have a good idea where you are.

Sample Conversation #1
You: What'll I do? What'll I do?
Best Friend: Why don't you just *talk* to him, for chrissakes?
You: What'll I say? I try to think of things to say, but I know I'll just end up sounding like a half-wit. What if he hates me? What if he already has a girlfriend?
　　Analysis: A crush. Note fear element.

Sample Conversation #2
Y: God, he was so cute! I couldn't believe it! With pectorals to die from, I swear. Speaking of pectorals, I wonder what Frank's doing tonight.
BF: I saw Frank with Angela last night.
Y: Oh really? Was she wearing that awful red dress? I got a postcard from Kevin the other day. . . .
　　Analysis: Boy-craziness. Note short attention span.

Sample Conversation #3
Y: He is, of course, the most wonderful man alive.
BF: So why don't you marry him or something?
Y: Maybe I should. But then, of course, I'm not the marrying kind. And anyway, I'm young yet, who knows who I might meet next? But gee, he sure does kiss like a champ. I dunno.
BF: Any guy who kisses like a champ is not a guy to be taken lightly.
Y: Yes, but . . .
　　Analysis: Serious like. Note commitment reluctance.

Sample Conversation #4

Y: There I was, minding my own business, when all of a sudden this *vision* appeared on the horizon. I lost all interest in my eggs. Do you think he goes there every day?

BF: Did I tell you about that guy I met last Tuesday when—

Y: I could tell he was watching me. I think I'll go back there tomorrow. I'll have French toast.

    Analysis: Instant lust. Leave it.

Sample Conversation #5

Y: I'm so happy I could die.

BF: Don't die.

Y: I've never felt this way about anyone before.

BF: Yes you have.

Y: No, not like this. This has been the most fabulous two weeks of my life. Everything is so perfect. He's so marvelously tall. So terrifically tender. So quintessentially *je ne sais quoi.*

BF: Say what?

    Analysis: Infatuation. Note use of word "fabulous."

Sample Conversation #6

Y: So then he says to me, he says, "Well then, how about Thursday night?" I mean, doesn't this guy have any pride, or what? Is he stupid? Is he blind?

BF: Maybe he's encouraged by the fact that you saw him three nights last week.

Y: But I'm not fucking him. Doesn't he notice that I'm not fucking him?

BF: Why don't you just stop seeing him?

Y: Just as soon as he puts up my bookshelves, I will.

    Analysis: Hatred, simple yet complex.

Sample Conversation #7

Y: No, I wasn't doing anything really, just lying around masturbating.

BF: How was work today?

Y: I hardly got anything done. I was too hung over.

BF: Hung over on a *Tuesday?*

Y: I dunno, I felt kind of restless last night. . . .

    Analysis: Advanced horniness.

Sample Conversation #8
Y: Well, I'm all packed. All my garter belts, stockings, stilettos . . .
BF: Which means you're going to see Floyd while you're there.
Y: Too right, BF. I can hardly wait.
BF: Maybe he'll convince you to stay there this time.
Y: What? And leave Illinois? You must be mad.
> *Analysis:* Lukewarm love and plenty of it.

Sample Conversation #9
Y: So how are you today? How's the sore throat?
BF: Better, thanks. How was Marcia's party?
Y: Exactly as expected, except that Marcia has a new protégé. A poet with pink hair who kept talking about the beauty in dead flowers. Steve and I kept trying not to look at each other so we wouldn't start giggling.
BF: How *is* Steve?
Y: He looks devastating at the moment, massaging my feet. Steve, BF wants to know how you are, you old lizard.
> *Analysis:* Sounds like love. Keep all fingers crossed.

Sample Conversation #10
Y: I didn't mean to do it. I just couldn't help it. When he answered, I hung up.
BF: You call him at three in the morning and then *hang up?*
Y: Well, I didn't want to wake him or anything. I just wanted to make sure he was home. He said, "I think I'll turn in early tonight," and I didn't know what he meant. . . .
> *Analysis:* Extensive obsession. Please turn the page.

6

The Perils of Obsession

"When your phone don't ring, it'll be me."
—GEORGE JONES

You sit there and stare at it, willing it to ring. It stares back at you, baleful and recalcitrant, not ringing. You throw a plate at it. Still nothing. Shouting obscenities, although pleasant, produces no results. You sit, stare at it again, then suddenly begin to pray feverishly: "Please God, let him call me in the next five minutes and I'll never even look at cocaine again—not even a little freeze. Just this once, God, be a darling and make him call me, and I'll become a nun as soon as this relationship is over. I promise. And I will also never again look down on those poor wretches who wear aqua polyester and don't care. In fact, if he calls in the next five minutes, I'll buy an aqua polyester pantsuit, *double-knit*, and wear it every day for a week. One time offer, God, act now."

Still nothing. Evasion tactics are in order. You turn cool, nonchalant—the phone could split a gut ringing, you could care less. You whistle carelessly, hum tunelessly and twiddle your thumbs while staring aimlessly off into space—any space at all so long as it doesn't have a horrid nonringing thing in it.

The phone, unfazed, continues its Clint Eastwood imitation—

strong, silent, unnerving. You consider, in an instant of fury, ripping it out of the wall. It doesn't mind.

Is it laughing at you behind its grim exterior? Probably. You wouldn't put it past that shiny little bastard. Look at the way it's just sitting there, gleaming at you malevolently.

You'll show it. You take a tea cozy and cover it completely. V*oilà!* No phone, no problem.

But wait. What if it's under there ringing away? Off comes the cozy.

No ringing. At all. Not even your mother, who calls at least eight times a day.

The phone is undoubtedly out of order. You pick it up, there is a cleverly misleading dial tone. Not fooled for an instant, you know for a fact that eight people at least have called in the past half hour, all of whom have been told that "The number you have reached has been disconnected."

It's *too* obvious. So you phone your best friend. "Hi there, it's me. Listen, I think my phone is out of order, I'm expecting some very important . . . What? Is it *that* late? Well, I'm sorry but . . . you were? Really? Yes, I know *those* dreams, but . . . Oh, God. Warren Beatty? Where? You did? How many times? Jesus, I'm sorry. But listen. Now that I've ruined it anyway, could you just call me back, what the hell? . . .

"Hello? Well, I guess it's working after all. No, nobody in particular, it's just that I'm expecting . . . Well, no, I haven't heard from him. Well, yes, he did, and he hasn't. No, it's not that I'm hyper, it's, well, maybe I should start at the beginning. The day before yesterday I think it was, we went to . . . Oh. Okay. You're right. Sorry. Maybe if you close your eyes real fast and think of Warren you'll just pick up where you left off, okay, bye."

Silence. Booming, deafening silence. You need a beer, or several. The grocery store on the corner will close in approximately three minutes. The moment you leave the house, the phone will ring. Phones simply adore ringing in empty houses.

You take the receiver off the hook. Then slam it back on again, convinced it is about to ring.

No, it isn't. Off the hook again. You fly to the store, trying to hide your sunken, staring eyes from the cashier, who is loudly chewing gum and looks like the type who never thought about telephones ringing in her life. Hard-boiled. Probably strings men up by their thumbs if they don't call when they say they will.

Then you run back to the house on swift, sure feet. The phone looks so sweet and helpless lying there with its receiver face up. No one could tell that it has evil lurking in its soul. You replace the receiver, drink three beers in quick succession and hope you're not turning into a character in a Dorothy Parker story.

Should you take a shower? You could bring the phone into the bathroom. You and that phone are becoming inseparable. Maybe you should propose to it. Marry the phone, cut out the middleman.

But can you really hear it ring if you're in the shower? Yes. It's ringing. Now that your hair is all sudsy, it rings. You hop out of the shower, streaming water, wait for your stomach to get out of your throat, pray fiercely for a second, and answer. Coolly.

Hello. Oh. Hi. No, I just walked in. Have you been trying to call? I know I said I'd be home, but . . . Really? No kidding. No, just out with a friend.

It's pitiful.

And this (this!) is the purported happy ending. One waits four, five, six hours for the phone to ring, and it actually does. You're redeemed, life is real, life is a phone call that actually came. You can now go to bed, bubbling with your good fortune.

Absolutely pitiful.

Is there one single human out there who has not at one point in her life been so obsessed that the telephone ruled her life with a heavy hand?

I heard of a three-year-old girl once, in love with a four-year-old boy named Stephano. The phone would ring, the three-year-old would rush to it and breathlessly answer, then the light in her eyes would dull.

"Who is it?" her mama would ask.

"Not Stephano," the little girl would say bleakly, handing the phone over. In her life, a person was either Stephano or not Stephano, and if it was not Stephano, it was nobody. This is your basic, no-frills obsession.

We tell ourselves we're not obsessed, we're in love.

How You Can Tell It's Not Love

When you're in love, you don't feel that secret, hardly recognized but all-pervasive sense of doom. There is a certain jaunty confidence deep in your heart of hearts. And the Significant Other is clearly reciprocating your feelings and just as nervous as you are.

I'm telling myself I'm in love right now, even as I type this. Another goddamned cowboy. Long, lean, and rangy. With the sweetest overbite and the slowest smile on earth. Two teen-aged children, an ex-wife, and a girlfriend. Lives in Colorado.

I'm obviously brain-damaged. I'm sitting here, telling myself he'll move to New York and any minute now we'll be wandering down Fifth Avenue together hand in hand, shopping for emerald earrings.

I lie in bed at night, trying to remember what he actually looks like. But as soon as I get the mouth in focus, I lose the eyes. I think about all the sentences he uttered and try on different meanings. Wonder whether, if I had said or done something different, he would be here beside me right now. I track down and pinpoint missed opportunities. Compose and recompose fascinating postcards.

A Tentative Definition of Obsession

Obsession is the grisliest of emotions. It is a macabre, hideous, gruesome, and horrific combination of pain, fantasy, and longing. The obsessed person turns herself all morbid and miserable and turns the object of her obsession into a shining, blinding-white light. Messy. Silly.

Symptoms of Obsession

—The last thing you think about before falling asleep is Him. If you happen to wake up in the middle of the night and crave some orange juice (obsessed people are notoriously thirsty), by the time you've gotten halfway across the room and before you've tripped over the coffee table and sent an entire vase of daffodils sprawling, you will again be thinking deeply of Him. When you wake up in the morning, you feel fine for a millisecond, then His name comes flooding into your consciousness, bringing with it dark fears, dank dreams, deep despair.

—You're convinced that he somehow knows every sniveling, needy thought that passes through your brain.

—Your stomach is too nervous to let you eat.

—When a normal person is talking to you, you nod intelligently and hear not a word.

—Books suddenly become unreadable.

—You have elaborate fantasies involving dozens of long-stemmed roses, midnight plane flights, and poignant marriage proposals.

—You wish you could again enjoy the restful calm of an anxiety attack.

—You stare at movies with unseeing eyes, even movies starring Richard Gere, even when Richard Gere takes his shirt off and stares moodily at the camera.

—Since he is devoted to ice hockey, you've noticed that you've developed a strange fascination for the game, and will actually watch hockey games on TV when "Fawlty Towers" is on another channel. Even though you're not absolutely sure what a puck is.

—You start walking around his neighborhood instead of doing the laundry. Or even in the neighborhood you think he *might* frequent once in a while, since he once bought a pair of shoes there. (I have a friend who was once obsessed with a businessman from Cleveland. She took to lurking around Sixth Avenue in Manhattan, reasoning that if he *were* by any chance in New York, he would be down on Wall Street, and *everyone* knows that to get out of Wall Street you have to take a cab up Sixth.)

—You have rehearsed dozens of casual yet captivating lines in case you actually do run into him.

—If he lives out of town, you stare at street maps of his home town until you get dizzy and pass out.

—Even though your friends threaten homicide if you don't shut up, you can't. You just have to know what they think he meant when he said that he often found that he couldn't sustain a relationship. Was he trying to warn you, or was he just being modest?

PSYCHOLOGICAL RAMIFICATIONS

The terrifying fact about an obsessed human is that she lives in utter misery and in a state of enormous passivity and no one has asked her to. Her every move and thought seems to be activated by thoughts of *him*, and yet there is hardly a man living who has ever walked up to a woman and said, "Hi there, I'm for you, but if you want me to love you, you have to think about me constantly and quiver with fear during my every silence. Every thought of yours must be of me. You must wear your hair in a style I find pleasing. You must not wear shoes that I don't like. If you fuck up, fuck you."

If any man ever sauntered over to you and said that, you would, depending on temperament, either dissolve into helpless giggles or set upon him with a chain saw. Obsession is solitary madness, self-imposed suffering, a prison camp built for one.

Why do we do this?

Damned if I know. Someone obviously dropped us on our collective heads when we were babies.

Many theories have been proposed: The obsessed person hates herself and is a masochist. The obsessed person loves herself and is a narcissist. The obsessed person is afraid of being overwhelmed by another person and therefore chooses only those who won't love her. The obsessed person is still in the throes of an Electra complex. The obsessed person is turning her repressed anger inward. The obsessed person was bottle-fed. The obsessed person is a latent homosexual.

Who cares? All we know for sure is that obsession is no way at all to have a good time.

There are at least two kinds of obsession:

OBJECT-RELATED OBSESSION

There are some men in this world who are not very nice. They get their kicks from causing pain and are adept at pushing the very buttons that will render the obsession-prone girl helpless and stupid.

"I'll never forget Peter," my friend Cleo says. "I still have nightmares. My heart was continually clanging around in my throat. All I ever thought was, 'Where is he? Why isn't he calling? Who is he with?' It was as if I didn't exist unless he called me. Horrible stuff. And he did it on purpose, the slimy creep."

I remember Cleo well during her Peter period. She was, poor angel, insufferable. This alleged man was king of the sadists, which, in New York City, is a pretty hefty title. We're talking bringing other girls to her place and leaving provocative letters in obvious places. We're talking disappearing for weeks at a time and telling her her thighs made him want to retch.

Cleo would call everyone at 3 A.M. and cry. Once she took a butcher's knife and hacked up all his letters, only to realize that in her enthusiasm she had also laid waste to her passport, a twenty-dollar bill, and her Bergdorf Goodman charge card.

"Cleo, he's a creep!" we would all scream. "He's not even that cute! He wears his shirt collar up! He can't pronounce the word annihilate! You're cute! You're smart! You know the meaning of the word xenophobic and don't let on! You've got great tits!"

"Oh, Peter's really not so bad," Cleo would sob after he spent the night with another woman on the very day she had an abortion. "He just had a lousy childhood, that's all. His father was cruel to him."

I ask you. We put up with three years of this. We watched in horror as Cleo became bedraggled and meek, how her eyes raced around a room at a party, how she started cooking gourmet meals, how she started reading *Cosmopolitan* for tips. *Cosmopolitan!* Cooking! This is not to say that making the perfect hollandaise may not be fine for many girls, but Cleo is the sort who breaks out in hives at the sight of a wok.

One day Cleo almost lost her job. Her boss told her she was becoming petulant, lazy, spiteful, and always on the defensive. Also, he said, he couldn't understand why she kept mispronouncing the word annihilate.

"Wait a minute," Cleo said to him, "you're describing Peter, not me."

"No, I'm not."

"Oh, my God," Cleo said, and broke up with Peter the next day. Luckily she still wanted a good job more than a depraved boyfriend.

She perked up enormously in a relatively short period of time.

THE CURE FOR OBJECT-RELATED OBSESSION

Leave town for the weekend. Bring a pen and paper with you. Check into a motel or something. Spend your days carefully calculating the happy moments and unhappy moments of your last month. Do not cheat. At night, go out and get drunk. The next day, tabulate your results. If you have been unhappy more than 50 percent of the time, break it off.

Just like that. Bite the bullet. It will hurt like major surgery, but if you don't do it, you'll just waste away. Three months, three years, three decades will go by and you'll realize that you haven't been you at all, that a huge chunk of your sweet life has been stolen by a marauding bandit.

You will be lonely. You will cry. You will wish you had never been born. You will curse the fates. You will rush to the phone approximately twenty-seven times per day to call him and beg him to take you back.

But take your finger off that dial. The dread obsession is a mighty master, and takes no prisoners. If you want to destroy yourself, you can always become a heroin addict.

The Floating-Fantasy Obsession

There are some girls who, if they aren't in a mild tizzy of obsession, get fidgety, restless, and fretful. A sort of hit-and-run machine, this girl. She fantasizes for one fellow for a bit, and then when he doesn't pan out, she'll shift to another, just like that.

The Cure for Floating-Fantasy Obsession

You must go to Las Vegas, Nevada, and find your way somehow to Caesars Palace. Then ask a scantily clad cocktail waitress or a stony-eyed blackjack dealer to direct you to the statue of David.

When Michelangelo created the original David, he felt that making the statue a mere thirteen feet tall would suffice. But at Caesars Palace, they had bigger and grander ideas. David is eighteen feet tall and weighs over nine tons. They just got carried away, those Caesars Palace boys, much the way we do when obsessed. They have taken a thing of beauty and instead created something overwhelming, gaudy, tasteless, and unwieldy—simply by making it too large.

Especially stare at the Caesars Palace David's genital area. If you do it long enough, you can put yourself into a mild trance.

As soon as you feel yourself hypnotized, start giving your subconscious a few autosuggestions to set it straight on this obsession business. I suggest something similar to the following:

"Listen, subconscious," say silently to yourself (if you actually speak aloud, armed guards will cart you off to a grisly fate in the desert), "it's time you and me had a little heart-to-heart. You've got to stop pulling this obsessiveness, it's bad for business. Possibly, subconscious, you've noticed that hugely hideous statue over there. Take it all in. And now, just try and picture that large thing in our living room.

"Where would we put it? What would we do with it? You can't even hang hats on it.

"It's just too goddamned big. Our ceiling, although adequate, could never encompass such a statue. We'd have to cut a hole through the ceiling, at which time our upstairs neighbors, nice people that they are, would turn snitty.

"We don't want the goddamned statue, do we, subconscious? Not on your life. And here we've been, turning nice, ordinary mortal men into virtual replicas of the thing.

"So, whaddya think? What say we reduce men to their normal size so that they'll fit into our life?"

Slowly count backward from five to one, and bring yourself out of the trance.

WHY BOTHER?

"So what?" you may think. "My obsessions might be a bit unrealistic, but at least they keep life perky. I mean, what else do I have to do with my time, take up needlepoint? How can a little obsession here and there hurt me?"

It's like this. Say you're obsession-prone and you meet a guy. Nice guy. Smart, funny, pleasant to be around, friendly, warmhearted. Maybe from Colorado or somewhere.

You become mildly interested in this guy, he feels likewise. You begin to cast secret speculative glances at each other, you wondering what kind of kisser he is, him thinking he sort of likes your crooked teeth although they may not be every man's cup of tea.

And then obsessiveness strikes, and you start thinking of him while ironing your hankies. You go out dancing and wish that he would walk through the door.

And then, when he *does* walk through the door, it's as if someone has shot a revolver very close to your left ear. Your throat gets dry, your heart pounds, you can't act normal.

A girl in this state does one of two things: too much, or not enough.

If she's an aggressive sort of girl, she'll act up. She'll watch him constantly, laugh a bit too loudly at his jokes, try to captivate him by talking a blue streak, and agree with everything he says. Each gesture and every word will be intensified beyond normalcy.

A man notices this intensity, and it puts him off. "Why is this nice girl suddenly acting like a nut case?" he asks himself.

No one except an actual sadist likes to be the object of an obsession. It makes a person nervous and jumpy and constantly wanting to look over his shoulder to see what all the fuss is about. Soon the object of an obsession will realize, and rightly so, that this sudden massive attention has nothing to do with him at all. He will become moody and distant, and that will be that.

If a girl is meek, yet obsessed, she'll suddenly become all quiet and scared, again way out of proportion, and the fellow will wonder if she's turned to stone or what. He used to tell her jokes and she used to laugh, he liked that. But now she just sits there and stares at him like he's a Martian. She used to be all sinuous and responsive when they danced, and now she keeps stepping on his feet and smashing her forehead into his nose. Where has the goddamned girl *gone*, anyway? Doesn't she like him anymore, or what?

When you're obsessed, you can't act normal, like the lovable old self who deserves to be loved.

(Quick here, before anybody gets the wrong idea, I want to point out that men get into this sort of fix just like women do. This is not a sex-related characteristic. At all. We've all had men being obsessed with us, and look where it got them.)

An obsessed girl may fall in love, she may get laid occasionally, but never as much as she would if she could just keep things in perspective.

A QUICK QUIZ TO TELL IF YOU'RE OBSESSED OR NOT,
JUST IN CASE YOU DON'T KNOW:

Envision yourself having this dialogue with the suspect:

You: What I'd really like to do is take a trip around the world
this summer.
Him: I wouldn't do that if I were you.
You: You wouldn't? Why not?
Him: Because you'd fall off the edge.
You: Edge? Edge of what?
Him: The world. It's flat.
You: Ha ha. No, what's the real reason?
Him: I'm quite serious. The world, as we know it, is flat. You
mustn't even *consider* taking a trip around it, since you will inevi-
tably fall off the edge and die.

Having got to this point in your conversation, would your response to his last statement be

(a) No it's not, you stupid git.

(b) Gee, I never knew that. How fascinating.

If you answered (a) you're fine. If you answered (b) you're not.

7

Sex Tips #2– Getting Acquainted

Q. Should you sleep with a man on the first date?
A. No, you should not.

No matter that he crushes you at your door in an embrace so mighty and flattening that you inadvertently buzz every doorbell in your apartment building. No matter that he falls to his knees and grasps the hem of your skirt, sobbing and pleading and promising rubies. No matter that you've worshipped him from afar since you were twelve. No matter that you haven't had an ounce of sex since the spring before last and you're afraid you'll dry up. No matter that he's just won the Nobel Peace Prize. No matter that he says he has a fatal disease and will definitely die by 10 A.M. the next day. Even if he promises to halt all nuclear-weapons activities, *don't do it*.

This is a hard-and-fast rule. There are no exceptions.

Except if you really want to.

I remember once, actually twice, okay, three times, when I did. The first time I ended up living with him for three years (that was Brian—three years of finding other girls' panties littering the apartment—what could I have been thinking?). The second was a sweet little guy at work who I just hadn't the heart to refuse. The third was my beloved and departed Jake.

In each case, it just seemed right. There we were, jabbering away like magpies, giggling and laughing and telling each other about the time when we were seven and found out for sure that only girls had vaginas, and it seemed the most natural thing in the world, as we were still giggling and talking at 5 A.M., as dawn crept over the city and the birds began having their own jolly chats, to simply fall into each other's arms. I remember thinking, What the hell.

But, come to think of it, these were guys that I knew before. I had worked with them, or seen them at my favorite restaurant all the time, or something. In one case I happened to be out of town, which, as everyone knows, doesn't count.

However, in ninety-nine cases out of a hundred, it is much more sensible to hang on a while until you feel comfortable and happy with the idea. Soulmates usually do not manifest themselves with alarming rapidity.

Here's another rule, and this time, no kidding around, no exceptions. Never, under any circumstances, ever go to bed with a man you've just met in a bar. Or any man you hardly know. No matter what.

Sleeping with a man you hardly know is like reading the end of a murder mystery first.

Sleeping with a man you hardly know is like eating a semiripe persimmon.

Sleeping with a man you hardly know is like licking the salty rim of the glass but forgetting to drink the margarita.

Sleeping with a man you hardly know is like eating freshly baked bread with a head cold.

It will be a stupid, stultifying experience. Even if he's Warren Beatty. Especially if he's Warren Beatty. Have you heard the same stories about Warren Beatty that I have? Sure you have.

ONE SHOULD BE A SEX MANIAC, BUT ONE SHOULD NEVER BE INDISCRIMINATE

Eventually you'll find that the time is right. You've been out with him a couple of times—the zoo, the movies, dinner, mud wrestling, and you've noticed a certain electricity every time your fingers touch. Salacious thoughts begin to occur, and you figure, Why not sleep with him before you go out of your mind with desire? A crucial moment, of course, but one with which every right-minded girl realizes she must contend. One must set the stage, let the man know how you feel, inform him of your eagerness to jump him. You can't, after buzzing him into your apartment, just lie there with your legs open and your eyes closed—it isn't seemly or kind. A bit of scene-setting is in order. Here are some tips:

—Start early. Get dinner or whatever over with by 10 P.M. at the latest, especially if one of you has to work in the morning. Better if neither of you has to work in the morning. Better yet to dispense with dinner altogether. You can always order a pizza.

—If the inevitable is going to happen at your house, don't riddle the house with candles and put mood music on the stereo. Candles and mood music are seduction clichés, and nothing puts a fellow off his feed so much as being the object of a textbook seduction. (Look at Sue Ann Nivens on "The Mary Tyler Moore Show." She never got anywhere.)

"Aha," a fellow thinks to himself, "look at all those candles. I bet she's planning to seduce me." The knowledge that he was also planning to seduce *you* will flee from his mind completely. He'll start feeling pressured, delicate flower that he is. And nervous, just like you. It's better if only one of you is a bundle of tortured ganglia.

—Never cook anything fancy like *pâté en croûte* or lobster Newburg. Even broiled grapefruit may be pushing it. Nothing makes a girl more annoyed than spending too much time in the kitchen. You'll start out thinking the absolute world of a fellow, but after a few hours with a pastry blender he'll begin to pale. "Who does he think he is," you'll start thinking to yourself, "making me sweat over a hot stove just to get into his pants? Does he think he's some kind of *gift* to women, or what? Well, the hell with him. I'm going to a movie instead." And then where will you be? Munching greasy popcorn and watching somebody else getting laid.

—Make sure you kiss someone before you go to bed with him. Pay careful attention. Does he thrust his tongue down your throat as if he's searching for the Holy Grail? Does he mash his teeth against your lips? If so, drop him flat. A man who can't kiss can't fuck. A proper kiss should be rife with sensitivity and playful in its sensuality. The tongue should be applied sparingly but with vigor. A bit of lower-lip nibbling is fine.

—If you're nervous, play a little Scrabble. Scrabble, being both boring and funny, is perfect for your purposes. During one of those tedious moments when he keeps shuffling his tiles around, you can grab him by his hair and tickle him. And by the time you get into a heated argument about whether or not hangup is really a word (it's not, and if it is, it shouldn't be), you'll find your nervousness vanished.

My friend Kate professes to be so shy that she has trouble talking to her mother. She has no reason to be shy, since she's cute, smart, bighearted and brimming over with the meanest wit this side of the Mississippi, but there you are. So Kate fell in love with Hank, a vaguely shy guy himself.

(Don't forget this: Any man who thinks of you as a living, breathing human and not an inflatable doll will be shy and insecure. He doesn't want to be rejected either.)

"If you're both shy," says Kate, "then you have to wait until it's time to say goodnight. Give him the greatest kiss in your repertoire and then just keep your arms around him, your pelvis gently pressed to his. Just leave it there, until you feel a familiar rising in his trousers, then kiss him again.

"You know," said Kate, digressing, "I remember going to dances when I was thirteen and wondering what that lumpy thing pressing against my stomach was. Was it his belt buckle? And if it was his belt buckle, why did he want to press it into me so much?

"Anyway, when a guy's shy and it takes you both a really long time to get to bed, then it's usually great when you get there. So I just keep on kissing him until neither of us has any choice."

Cleo, who's a bit more aggressive, has been known to say, "If you don't press your body up against me right this minute, I'll probably die." She promises it works.

So then you go to bed. For many girls, this is pure, unadulterated bliss.

"But not for me," says Kate, back among us. "I just can't get over the fact that this person is going to see my naked body. I think about my ass, which is fat but doesn't look so bad with clothes on. I get so self-conscious! And also, this is an awful thing to say, but I feel like there's an intruder in my bedroom. Almost like, oh, this is *stupid* but almost like this perfectly normal guy has turned into an enemy.

"Anyway, I've only had three boyfriends before. I'm not some kind of swinging, liberated chick. And I guess I don't trust anyone very much."

And who can blame her? Not me, not you. If I know you, you're no virgin. You've had your share of broken promises, devastating misunderstandings, heartbreaking phone calls, stony breakfasts, smashed crockery and ego battering.

After all this, it is a tremendous act of faith for any girl to whip off her clothes and expose herself, naked and alone, in front of a new man. To take that great transcendental leap of faith yet again. Makes you think you've lost your marbles even contemplating it.

Of course, there are girls who fuck people all the time and think nothing of it. But these girls, I have it on good authority, don't trust any man. They tell themselves they're looking for Mr. Right, but such haphazard behavior makes them feel rotten about themselves and leads them inevitably into the arms of Mr. Wrong. They turn defensive and hard.

But if you have even a soupçon of vulnerability left, you're going to be deeply frightened the first time.

Do a bit of deep breathing. Put your favorite record on. Go into the bathroom and have a little deep communion with your diaphragm. Look at yourself in the mirror and admire the way your hair curls so adorably. And then go pay attention to the man in the other room.

He's out there, wandering around the living room, pretending to study your bookshelves and wondering if he should go into the bedroom or what. "Is she the kind of girl who'll want me to undress her?" he's asking himself. "Will we have oral sex first?"

He's got his eyes closed tight, trying his damndest to remember how big his penis is. He *thought* it was pretty big when he put on his terrific new sky-blue boxer shorts earlier this evening, looked to be about seven or eight inches, maybe even nine. But who knows? Maybe it shrunk. Maybe it looks just like a peanut now.

Ah, there you are now, finally emerging from the bathroom, grinning at him playfully. This playful grin is precisely what he needs right now. A grin that says, "Peanut for a penis or not, you're a hell of a guy and I want to jump you."

Expert opinion varies widely on this. But many don't believe in tearing off your clothes and leaping straight into bed. The first night is a good night for prolonged foreplay. Let him toy with your nipples a lot. When he tries to put his hand under your skirt, wriggle away a little. (This is a turn-on for both of you—the wriggle itself is lust-provoking, and pretending to elude his grasp will make you remember those steamy nights in high school after the basketball game.)

Toy with him. Rub your fingertips gently along his thighs and knees, never actually touching his penis but acting as if you might any second now. This kind of teasing will dispel any fears he has about his penile size—he'll get so excited he'll feel like John Dillinger.

Meanwhile, you'll be playing around with your tongue, lightly tracing squiggles around his ear, darting it jauntily into his mouth for a moment and licking his front teeth.

When you finally touch him, try sincerely not to act like one of those ladies in the supermarket testing peaches. The most sensitive parts of the penis are right along the rim of the tip and that ridge that runs down the back of it. Take your fingers and massage these parts gently but firmly. Don't giggle.

How you actually get into bed is your own affair. The ideal way, of course, would be to have Scotty to beam you in, but somehow Scotty is never there when you need him. Many girls simply opt for dragging a man by his belt buckle. Lacks finesse, but gets the job done. If it's *his* apartment, let him take the lead.

Now that you're in bed, pay serious attention. Look at the fellow next to you, notice the way his neck curves into his shoulder, the way his bicep bulges against your pillow, the way his erection presses against you.

Don't show off. There's nothing more daunting to a man in the throes of passion than to have his partner suddenly turn into a trapeze artist. Even if you are proficient in chinning yourself on the curtain rod while simultaneously throwing your buttocks to a flamenco rhythm, try to save those pyrotechnics for later. You don't want to shoot your wad (sorry) on the first night, and erections have a way of shrinking when confronted with circus acts.

And speaking of erections, have you thought about them lately? No, really. An erection is caused by all the blood which is usually housed in the brain suddenly deciding to desert the gray matter and settle in the penis, which is why a man can't think and fuck at the same time. (Yogi Berra once said, in a moment of blinding insight, that he just couldn't think and hit at the same time. Which proves, once and for all, that he is a Zen master.)

Erections. Caused by that most vital and tenuous fluid, blood. Which means that many things can go wrong, since the brain often gets furious at the blood's desertion and decides to fight back. There a man will be, lying there happily with an erection as big as the Ritz, and suddenly the brain will strike a devastating blow.

"Did you remember to deduct that trip to Kalamazoo on your tax return?" the brain will taunt the poor unsuspecting fellow. "Isn't today your sister's birthday? Did you mail the check for your fishing license? Did you remember to lock your car?"

Next thing the poor guy knows, all the blood has rushed back to the brain again. His erection is a thing of the past. A dead issue. History.

And you can't fake an erection. So, just for a moment here, let's all join hands and thank the Lord that we're not men—that we never in our whole long and lovely lives have to worry about the up-keep and care of erections.

To show how grateful you are, you must promise never to aid and abet performance anxiety. Your average man is exceedingly sensitive about his masculine image, and it sometimes gets to the point where he forgets about having a good time, he's so goddamned nervous. Plus he's read all those books and articles and knows for sure that you are expecting the cosmos to move with the very first twitch of his tongue on your clitoris. You, he assumes, are an exacting sort of girl, not one to be content with any prosaic breast-fondling. You want him to go the *Kama Sutra* one better.

Poor bastard, if he only *knew*. Most of us would kiss the ankles of a man who lets his passion overtake him to the point where he forgets all the amenities. Call us weird, but we love that. Passion—the feeling that a man wants us so badly he can hardly breathe—is the ultimate aphrodisiac.

Let him know this. But use finesse; it won't do to simply say, "Cut the crap and let's fuck."

You may, if you're the verbal type, say something along the lines of "God, I'm so excited that if you even bite my earlobe again I'll probably come."

But if you're too shy to say stuff like this, the body is an eloquent organ with a language all its own, and it has no irregular verbs like Latin or Portuguese.

Here are some simple body sentences and their English translations. Study them carefully. There will be a pop quiz at the end of the chapter.

BODY SENTENCE

Take his hand, put it on your breast and simultaneously nibble his earlobe.

TRANSLATION

There's something about you that drives me into paroxysms of quivering passion. Take me right now.

BODY SENTENCE

Put his finger into your mouth and suck on it suggestively.

TRANSLATION

There's something about me, I don't know exactly what, that makes me want to suck on things, although this finger isn't completely satisfying. Perhaps you'd like to suggest an alternative?

BODY SENTENCE

Encircle his ankle with your hand and run your tongue along the circumference of his navel.

TRANSLATION

If we don't do it in the next thirty seconds I'll probably die.

BODY SENTENCE

While he's lying on his back, straddle him and insert his penis inside you.

TRANSLATION

Hello there, sailor.

See how easy?

FIRST NIGHT IMPOTENCE

Sometimes a man loses his erection and can never get it back, and sometimes, funnily enough, he just can't get an erection at all.

Impotence is one hell of a note. But one must keep one's sense of humor. One mustn't get rattled or impatient.

What one must not do, no matter what, is to keep kneading the penis as if one were preparing dinner rolls. This will only make him sad. Also refrain from saying wistfully, "Do you think it will go up soon?" This is an excruciating moment for a man, and the only thing to do with anything excruciating is to ignore it. Be light and airy, be devil-may-care.

Say something like "Don't be silly, it doesn't matter. I'm just glad to be here with you, and you looked so dashing tonight in that white boat-necked sweater. God, that reminds me, you know what happened to me yesterday? A grown man in a sailor suit walked up to me, told me he was an extraterrestrial, and demanded to be taken ice-skating."

"Really?" he'll say, and before you know it, you'll be immersed in discussion. Why ice-skating? Why a sailor suit? Was this a come-on? An extraterrestrial courting ritual?

And there you'll be, having a good time and letting his quiescent erection nurse its battered self-image. Maybe he'll eventually get it up, maybe he won't. First-night impotence is a widespread phenomenon, and nothing much to worry about. (Long-termed, prolonged impotence over several weeks, months or years is a different story and will be taken up in a subsequent chapter.)

ORGASMS, CARE AND FEEDING OF

So what about you already? What about *your* fears, *your* performance anxiety? Okay, maybe you don't have to have an erection, but you do have to have an orgasm, don't you? What will he think if you don't have an orgasm? He'll probably think you're some sorry excuse for a female. He'll probably think you're a neurotic sicko of the first order. He'll probably think you're frigid and also a lesbian.

There you go, getting yourself all worked up, all in a dither. And for what?

Many, maybe most, women don't come the first time they sleep with a man. And nobody can make you have an orgasm when you don't want to, even you.

But women will often try. We'll clench our teeth, squinch our eyes shut and think, "I will have an orgasm! I will! I will!"

Your body takes umbrage at this sort of authoritarianism. Not only will it not give you an orgasm, it will make you feel like a fool.

Leave your body alone. Trust it, give it its space. Yours is not to reason why, let alone do or die.

It is permissible to ask the fellow next to you for help. What, after all, are friends for? Again, use finesse. Don't stare at him reproachfully if he doesn't get it right the first time.

And many guys will not get it right. They often think of the clitoris as if it were a teensy penis, and treat it as such. A penis, as we know, actually craves a good deal of pressure, but the clitoris, as we also know, is a sensitive, elusive little devil. If you touch it directly, it hurts. You have to kind of sneak up on it.

When a man does it right, say, "I love that." When he does it wrong, distract him with an amusing anecdote.

My friend Cleo told me an interesting story.

"I had a cataclysmic breakthrough a while ago," Cleo said. "A man was massaging my clitoris at the time. And I was enjoying it. In fact, I was loving it."

"So what else is new?" I asked.

"I didn't always," Cleo confided. "I used to be wretchedly ashamed that I even *had* a clitoris. The idea that it could actually give me pleasure seemed degrading. When a guy touched it, I wanted to hide under my pillow. Know what I mean?"

"Sure."

"But this time, I felt like I was a kid again, before I knew this stuff was bad. Oh, I knew it was *naughty*, but not really bad, you know? Anyway, it was like me and James were two little brats, two co-conspirators, doing something a little naughty but a lot of fun. And suddenly James wasn't some guy I was trying to impress with my rampant sensuality. We were in it together. It was great."

Woody Allen was right when someone asked him if he thought sex was dirty and he said, "If you do it right." Sex is not some sort of pristine, reverent ritual. You want reverent and pristine, go to church. You want to cure first-night jitters? Pretend you're playing doctor.

There is one thing you should never do, no matter how much you want to. You must never fake an orgasm. Faking an orgasm is an act of self-degradation, and it sets up a behavior pattern that ruins your self-esteem, gives you anxiety headaches, and destroys your faith in humankind. If you fake an orgasm, you're wreaking havoc with your karma.

Sometimes this is a very hard thing not to do. There you both are, you've been at it for at least two hours and you can tell your partner is dying to come, but he's too much the gentleman to do it until you do. But you can't. You're worried about how you're going to afford that trip to Italy, or whether you should quit your job, or maybe your body is just being perverse. And you figure, Why not put the poor fellow out of his misery and fake it.

Well if you must, you must, but don't. Sexual satisfaction is based on trust, and every faked orgasm is a lie, one more barrier between the two of you.

You'll have to tell him sooner or later, or you'll start resenting him. Sooner is better.

Say something like, "Please don't hold back on my account. My body is not behaving." No need for choked confessions or flowery speeches.

There will be no pop quiz as threatened. Instead, here's a Richard Pryor joke:

MAN: Baby, I think your pussy's dead.

WOMAN: Well, why don't you give it mouth-to-mouth resuscitation?

8

Sexual Etiquette

"What do we do now?" everyone is constantly asking.

In the old days, those primordial times before the sexual and feminist revolutions, etiquette between the sexes was a cinch. We knew exactly what was expected of us—let the man pay the check, wait by the telephone for the man to call, tell the man no when we meant yes. (If we really meant no, we'd have to rake his cheek with a scarlet fingernail.)

But nowadays you can't even walk to the corner without encountering clusters of earnest women debating on what the hell the male species is up to and what we're supposed to do about it.

"Should I call him?" we wonder, "or shall I wait for him to call me? If I wait for him to call me, how long should I wait? Three days? Three months? And if he doesn't call me after three months, should I call him then? If I do break down and call him, what should I say? How do I do it so that I don't sound like an imbecile? Should I care about sounding like an imbecile? Am I an imbecile?

"Then again, what if he does call and invites me to dinner? Should I insist on paying the check? Should I quickly go and powder my nose when the check comes?

"Or should we split the check? If he pays, does that mean I have to put out? If I pay, can I make him iron my shirts? Who sends the flowers? What flowers?"

It's a nightmare, a true morass of manners. But it could be a lot worse. Cast your mind back to those horrifying days when all we wanted were white dresses and wedding veils.

We are now in the enviable position of having a clean slate. Since nobody knows what the hell is going on, we are in the position to get in on the ground floor, etiquettewise. We can write the book. Who can stop us?

Herewith I would like to propose the new laws of sexual etiquette. The chair will entertain motions from the floor.

TELEPHONE MANNERS

—*On phoning a man you hardly know:*

When in doubt, blunder ahead. A woman may call a man any time she feels like it.

Do not rehearse long speeches. No fellow likes to answer the phone and hear, "Hi! It's me, Jean. We met at Helen's party, remember? Well, I was just watching 'Family Feud' and it reminded me of that funny thing you said about your mother. God, that was really hilarious. I just thought I'd die laughing. Old Helen sure knows how to give a party, although she didn't used to. You probably won't believe this, but two years ago, Helen used to serve the rumaki *after* dessert. I was too embarrassed to tell her, but somebody did. I think it was Chrissie. Speaking of Chrissie, there's a great movie at the NuArt tonight, *The Americanization of Emily.* It doesn't *seem* like it would be any good but it is. Wanna go?"

Now, there's nothing actually *wrong* with the above, except possibly the imperfect transition between the rumaki and the NuArt. But a fellow does sometimes like to get a word in edgewise, dazzling a girl with his off-the-cuff wit and so forth, and this sort of rehearsed speech doesn't give him a chance. Plus you'll be so worried about getting your lines right you won't notice his bons mots.

—*Proper preparations for calling a man:*

1. Have a vague purpose for the call. You don't want to start trailing off into "Um, well, yes . . . I just thought I'd call. I don't know, I just thought . . ."

2. Get in a friendly frame of mind. So many girls, deciding on the assertive measure of picking up the phone, go the whole hog and segue right over into aggression. They get so scared that a man is going to think, "What's this moron calling me for?" that they go off their heads, making the giant paranoiac leap to being convinced that he does, for sure, think she's a moron, and not a very attractive moron at that. When he finally picks up the phone, she says "Okay, so I'm a moron, so what? Wanna go to the movies with me or not? Think you're too good for me, you jerk?"

Even if the fellow doesn't quite remember you, he'll be totally delighted to get your call. It's nice for his ego, makes him think he's a pretty sharp fellow, having girls call him. This will make him chatty.

—*On phoning a man you've slept with recently but don't know where you stand:*

It used to be, back in less convoluted days, that if a man didn't call you the afternoon after spending the night, you were in deep trouble.

Now, after a couple spends the night together, both of them are in deep shock. What have they done? What are the ramifications of this sexual tryst? Is it meaningful? Is it a relationship? Is it just a shallow, pointless one-nighter? Should they keep Saturday night open? How about New Year's Eve? How about never mind?

Things are so fraught and confusing that many people just say fuck it and give up. Especially men. At present, men are emotionally more cowardly than women.

Give him a breathing period, and then call him just to say howdy.

One must not use undue pressure, however. If he acts cool and remote, do not call him again, unless it's to say that he's a maladjusted toad for toying with your affections like that.

—*More telephone hints:*

It is not proper to call a man during the Super Bowl, during the Kentucky Derby, during a World Series game, or during the Stanley Cup games. No, not even during halftime or between innings or periods, when he is invariably on the phone with his bookie talking point spreads.

—Do not call a man more than twice in one day, unless to impart crucial information, like that the movie isn't at 8:10 after all, but at 7:45. Or that your house just caught fire and if he wants his records he'd better hop to it. If you call a man three times in one day just to ask him what he had for lunch or why the sky is blue, you tend to lose your mystery.

—Do not fight over the telephone.

—Do not say "Hi, it's me" when you call a man, without identifying yourself further. This can lead to confusion, even unpleasantness.

—One should not answer the telephone during sex, even if it might be your agent.

—One should spend no more than five minutes, ten minutes tops, on the phone while entertaining a hot prospect. And never get cute and start whispering into the receiver with a seductive throatiness when another man is in the room.

—Call a man at three in the morning only after you've known him for at least three months. Never call a man at four in the morning unless he's been threatening suicide.

—Do not accept phone calls from men who say, "Hi, it's me."

ANSWERING SERVICES

If you use an answering service, get as friendly as possible with the operators. Bribe them if necessary. Otherwise they'll let your phone ring fifteen times before deigning to answer, or they'll lose any message that might sound promising and only give you those from your mother. Sometimes, if an operator is feeling downright sadistic, she'll make things up. Answering-service operators have been known to tell an unsuspecting girl that her gynecologist called and said she's got the clap, or that Richard called and never wants to see her again.

If the man you're calling has an answering service, always tell the operator that you're Diane Keaton or Candice Bergen. All operators are dreadful snobs, and like to shield their clients from anyone they consider riffraff.

ANSWERING MACHINES

It is not necessarily clever to record clever messages on your answering machine. If you have your machine say, "Hi, this is Susan.

I took too many drugs last night and am now spending three hours in the shower trying to get my eyes to stay in my head. Please leave a message," the only people who will call are your seventy-four-year-old Aunt Clara, a bill collector, and your shrink. Answering machines have a secret connection with the cosmos and can effect things like that.

When speaking to a Significant Other's machine, don't worry about sounding like a pinhead. Everyone does. Best to just say your name and number and hang up quickly before you do irreparable damage to your self-image.

WHAT IS A DATE?

A date, at this juncture in history, is any prearranged meeting with a member of the opposite sex toward whom you have indecent intentions. A date in Manhattan usually involves going to nightclubs where everyone is dressed in black-on-black. A date in Los Angeles often entails sushi bars. A date in Texas means crossing the border into Mexico and coming home three days later remembering nothing. A date in Philadelphia means falling asleep in front of the TV together. A date in San Francisco means wondering if your date has had a sex change.

But you have to keep on your toes, because literally anything could turn into a date. Once a man asked me to walk him to his shrink, and halfway there I realized he was serious.

WHO PAYS?

You do, whenever you can. It's not just chivalry that makes a man grab the check from the waitress before anyone else does. He *likes* paying the check. It gives him a warm and wonderful feeling of power and well-being, knowing that the sweat of his brow just transmuted itself into several orders of moo goo gai pan. The frequency of check-paying should be determined by income, not sex.

One must not turn it into a production. Do not grapple a man to the floor or kick him and shriek, "Let me pay or your balls are in jeopardy!" since that's exactly what he's afraid of. Be gracious. If he insists on paying, let the sucker.

If you decide to split the check, split it down the middle. In this area, men have it all over women. You've seen women at lunch with their calculators ("Now Doris, you had the second Tab, so yours will come to $8.42. No, wait, I forgot the tax. Oh hell! Let's see— $8.76? I think that's right. No, wait, Daphne, you had the espresso. Hang on a sec. . . .") By the time everyone gets up to leave, a half-hour of valuable time later, each woman is convinced that she alone has overpaid for her less generous, more conniving friends. She feels cheated, disgruntled.

If a man is much wealthier than you are, still pay when you can. Even a man who's rich as Croesus will get a kick out of being treated occasionally. It makes him feel all pampered and sweet and taken care of.

One does not have to sleep with, or even touch, someone who has paid for your meal. All those obligations are hereby rendered null and void, and any man who doesn't think so needs a quick jab in the kidney.

GIFTS

One may always accept modest presents and feel no obligation, sexual or other.

But it is still bad form to accept expensive trinkets and then go whistling off into the night. A man may give you an emerald brooch because he has great respect for your keen sophisticated wit, and not simply because he wants to get into your pants. But if you accept that brooch, sweetheart, you must be prepared to put out. Only if you were going to anyway can you pin the sparkly little devil right to your lapel and say, "Thank you my darling Cecil."

But don't hold out for emerald brooches. That's just fancy prostitution, and besides you may find yourself enjoying long periods of celibacy—emerald brooches cost a mint. I personally have been hinting for years. Ask anyone.

One must buy a man gifts only out of generosity. Do not spring a diamond tie clasp on a man to make him feel guilty, or to get him to love you.

And one must never buy a man a Lear jet or anything else intimidating.

SPENDING THE NIGHT AT YOUR APARTMENT

Amy Vanderbilt says, "A girl who has a home to which a man may come and be entertained has a better chance than the siren who lives in a hotel room and must be taken continuously to meals, movies, theaters, and nightclubs. Such a girl costs too much and is too wearing. . . ."

If possible, move immediately to a hotel.

If you can't, make sure your home is reasonably clean and neat, but do not equip it unduly with video games and pool tables and indoor swimming pools or you'll never get to go to nightclubs.

But do keep your floors swept, your sheets pristine, and your bathtub free from any and all stray pubic hair. There should be no moldy dishes in the sink.

Never spend more than an hour and a half cleaning your apartment for a fellow. Four hours of waxing floors, polishing silver, and scrubbing toilets will make you resent even the most devastating of dreamboats. By the time the poor fellow arrives, you'll be seething.

"Hi, honey," he'll say.

"Oh, go fuck yourself," you'll answer snappily.

This is not a good start for a fun evening.

One should, however, have a thoughtfully stocked refrigerator. Several bottles of imported beer or a couple of bottles of decent wine are *de rigueur*. A few fancy snacks cooked up by a nearby gourmet shop will not go amiss—although, in a pinch, raisin bran will do fine.

It is always a pleasant and generous gesture to provide soft drugs for your guest. Sensemilla if one has the money and inclination, a couple of bottles of Nyquil if one does not.

Your bathroom should be free of aerosol shaving cream and jockstraps, unless you have a male roommate. And it is unforgivable, when Howie is visiting, to leave your diary opened conspicuously to a page which says "Dinner etc. with darling Freddie."

Remember, keep the candles to a minimum.

Do not, until you are utterly convinced beyond a shadow of a doubt that he wants them, offer a man keys to your apartment.

SPENDING THE NIGHT AT A MAN'S HOME

When taken to a man's home for the first time, it is not acceptable to shriek with dismay. Refrain from saying, "What a dump," unless his house is palatial *and* he is devoted to Bette Davis.

One must, instead, try to be a good sport, unless he has left a full kitty-litter box in the bathtub. Men, as a race, are notoriously bad housekeepers, but a man who leaves kitty litter in the bathtub is being actively insulting. ("The hell with it," you can almost hear him saying to himself, "why should I take the kitty litter out of the bath for some dumb broad?") This is a slap in the face, and must not be tolerated.

Other nonacceptable items in a man's domicile are obvious signs of another woman (unless he has a female roommate), dirty or stained sheets, or indications of severe drug abuse. So, if there are nail-polish bottles sitting on his bookshelves, malodorous sheets on the bed, or a syringe, spoon, and several glassine envelopes scattered about his kitchen table, call a taxi immediately.

Whips, handcuffs, or other exotic sexual paraphernalia should never be in evidence. If he should happen to possess such articles, a man must keep them entirely to himself until that unlikely day that a female companion actually requests them.

No man, however obsessed, may ever keep a paper bag full of garter belts under his bed and whip them out at a crucial moment, begging his partner to find one that fits.

No woman, however intimate with a man, may ever buy him new curtains, even if his existing ones are moth-eaten and crusted with dirt. Men get distinctly jittery about this.

Similarly, one should never wash a man's dishes. He will not be filled with gratitude and *joie de vivre* but will instead feel the noose closing around his neck. Men, being conditioned badly, are always feeling nooses closing around their necks, even dumpy boors no girl would take on a bet.

BREAKFAST

It is customary, unless one of you must get to work for an early meeting, to have breakfast *à deux* after spending the night together.

If at his house, the man must go to the grocery store to purchase eggs and bacon and such, while you lounge prettily in bed reading magazines. If at your house, you, regrettably, should go. Better yet, both of you hit the nearest coffee shop.

Some of the best men refuse to talk at breakfast and will spend the entire meal engrossed in the sports pages. Let him do this. There is no one surlier than a man who wants to find out if the Lakers won or not and can't.

LUNCH

Lunch is a meal you have with anyone you're not planning on sleeping with. Reserve it for your friends.

BELONGINGS

It is permissible, even advisable, to bring a small overnight bag when one is sure one is spending the night, but it is seriously problematical to show up one fine day with three suitcases and a birdcage.

When you leave in the morning, take everything with you. Yes, even your toothbrush. Leaving a change of clothes in the bottom drawer of his dresser, when not specifically invited to, is encroaching and presumptuous.

If a man starts leaving his socks around for you to wash and his after-shave perched coyly on your bathroom shelf, he's being possessive. Don't let him do this if you don't want him to. Just bundle up those socks and put them neatly into a fashionable shopping bag, then present the bag to him sweetly as he makes his way out of your door in the morning. Be friendly but firm.

OTHER RELATIONSHIPS

A person who regales her dinner date with exhaustive stories of her ex-husbands and ex-lovers is a person who doesn't know the meaning of the word discretion.

If you tell a man about the way your ex-husband used to call you his sweet patootie right before coming, or how your old boyfriend used to like it when you tied him to the drainpipe, a man may start to think things. He'll think, "What the hell will she say about *me* when we break up?"

If you *must* confide this sort of sexual memorabilia, confine yourself to one or two girlfriends who can keep their mouths shut.

If you are seeing more than one person, keep it to yourself until required to tell. If a man starts getting a wedding-bells look in his eye, or if he lets you know that it's only a matter of moments before the two of you set up housekeeping, the time is overripe for letting him know you're still playing the field.

If you're not seeing someone else but want a man to think you are, think again. "Making him jealous" is a game only to be played by teenagers. No man in his right mind puts up with a girl who keeps parading in front of his house with her exercise instructor.

NAME-CALLING

Whereas black people can call each other "nigger" with impunity, a white person may not presume to do so unless he doesn't mind dying.

Similarly, we can call each other girls, chicks, broads, birds and dames with equanimity. Many of us prefer to do so since the word "woman," being two syllables, is long, unwieldy, and earnest.

But a man must watch his ass. Never may a man be permitted to call any female a "chick." He may call you a broad or a dame only if he is a close friend and fond of John Garfield movies. The term "bird," generally used by fatuous Englishmen, is always frowned upon.

Sometimes the term "girl" is permissible, sometimes it isn't. Some men will use it with such condescension that you'll want to throttle them, whereas other fellows obviously don't have a smidgeon of malice aforethought. Although "girl" is never strictly proper, you may let these latter guys slide.

The term "gal," however, can never be tolerated except from Texans, to whom the term "good old gal" is actually high praise.

When offended by a sexist slur, do not fall to the floor, kick and scream and hold your breath. The cold freeze is much more dignified.

To effect the cold freeze, simply pretend you're a duchess. Arch one eyebrow disdainfully, point the nose distinctly skyward, and pronounce the word "Indeed" with chilling accents. Make sure that your eyes display rampant disapproval. (You may have to practice this look in front of the mirror. You'll know you've got it right when the mirror breaks into pieces and slinks to the floor.)

Then turn loftily on your heel and beat it.

GAME-PLAYING

> "*When in doubt, tell the truth.*"
> —Pudd'nhead Wilson

Although we shouldn't, we all play games. Games as in manipulation. These can range in severity and complexity from the relatively simple "Not tonight dear, I have a headache" to the mind-boggling "If you really loved me, you wouldn't become a neurosurgeon."

We're all cunning little sods, and we play these games every chance we get. If someone happens to call us on it, we say, "Game? Me? Whatever *are* you talking about? I merely said . . ." And we mean it, because we don't know we're doing it. No, really, we don't. Honestly.

It's that nasty unconscious again, making words come out of our mouths, we know not why. Probably when we were three years old, we happened to overhear our mothers say, "Darling, Jack Ames says I look lovely in my new dress."

To which Dad grunted, "That's nice dear, pass the potatoes."

"Jack's such a good husband, don't you think?" Mom continued.

"You should have married *him*," Dad said.

"No need to take that tone with me, Harold," Mom said. "I merely said . . ."

Now you were only three years old at the time and too busy sticking your mashed bananas up your nose to really pay attention, but your unconscious was pricking up its ears, all right. So now, a grown-up adult, you play approximately thirty-seven games a day and don't even know it. But if you happen to catch yourself at it, stop it. In mid-sentence, if necessary.

The biggest game in town, male-femalewise, is the game called "I don't care as much about you as you do about me." This singularly unappealing game is spreading like wildfire in major metropolitan areas. Girls tell men they have another dinner engagement when they really don't. Guys tell girls they don't want a commitment when they're really just scared.

It is an endless dance in which the participants just go around in circles until they drop from exhaustion and confusion.

The motive behind the game is self-protection. There is nothing wrong with this in theory; people must protect themselves. But sometimes they get so carried away that they think everyone is an enemy, and resort to war tactics and retaliations before any outbreak of hostilities. Which just leaves everyone lonely, depressed, and afraid.

My friend Kate is a sweet newlywed who not only will listen to my unceasing problems but will also often throw some useful advice my way.

On the day in question, I was complaining that a man I'd been seeing broke a date with no explanations.

"What shall I do?" I said. "Should I refuse to see him anymore? When he calls, should I act all pert and jolly and keep putting him off when he wants to see me? That should make him paranoid. Maybe I'll pretend I've fallen in love with someone else. Maybe I'll wait outside his door all night and scratch on it pathetically at 7 A.M."

"And then when he opens it," she said, "you can say, 'Oh please oh please oh please love me.' Attach yourself to his ankles and grovel."

"That's it!" I cried. "Pleading and begging! Brand-new method for getting a man to be nice to you!" But then I got depressed again. "No, really. What should I do? Should I act like I don't care?"

"Well," said Kate, "this may sound stupid, but I think people should always tell the truth. A lot of times it's easier to lie, and sometimes it seems to work out better when you do, but it doesn't, really. You don't want someone to care about you for all the wrong reasons."

We decided, then and there, that only brave people tell the truth, and only brave people get what they want.

9

Sex and the Single Parent

Now that he's getting older, I've been trying to convince my son to start calling me Auntie. But he won't. Children are like that and, although living with them has unimpeachable rewards, a child's dogged demand for honesty, integrity, and someone to flip baseball cards with can turn the single woman's life into a living, breathing sitcom.

There are a lot of us single parents running around these days. We got married, had a kid or two, realized we had opted for domesticity a bit too soon, and decided to hit the streets.

Only to find, of course, that domesticity followed us everywhere, like the dim-brained but faithful puppy who trotted along to school every day.

Nonetheless, it's great fun having a kid around, since then you don't have to explain to anyone why you have a full-size poster of Reggie Jackson in the living room or why you've seen *Star Wars* five times.

The first thing every single parent must do is keep a meticulous diary. You will soon have enough material for five stirring, poignant screenplays simply oozing with cuteness, and can easily become a millionaire and never have to do your own laundry again.

"I want three limousines, a ranch with fifty horses, and several airplanes," my son told me when I detailed these plans to him.

The second thing you must do is resign yourself to a semi-demented sex life. For the single parent, having a sex life is much like trying to climb Mount Everest in a cocktail dress. One wants to make it look simple and effortless, but those telltale beads of sweat keep forming on the upper lip.

Confusions are rampant. Is it a good idea to keep your children and your men completely separate? Should you try, right off the bat, to bring your latest love into the family circle? Should you be happy when your kid and your man become enmeshed in a week-long game of Dungeons and Dragons? What if your kid punches your fellow in the solar plexus? What if your fellow buys your kid a drum kit?

And what if they hate each other? And how dare you go out on dates anyway? What kind of mother are you? A rotten one? Shouldn't you be constantly at home, nurturing?

Nobody said it was going to be easy. But it's not too hard, and it's always funny. You simply have to sort out a few problems.

GUILT

Scratch a single parent (and not too hard) and you will tap a mother lode of guilt. The litany goes like this: You, single parent, have to be both mother and father to the darling tyke. You must not only bring home the bacon but also be there to kiss and make better skinned knees and smashed toenails. Your child is deprived and bereft, so you must keep your nose to the old grindstone. It is sinful to go to parties, let alone take a midnight swim or two, and if you do so, you are a bad person.

The only thing to do with parental guilt is laugh loudly in its face until it realizes how ridiculous it is and slinks away. Of course you're supposed to have a good time! You're not dead, are you?

Kids have been known to play on this guilt, since kids, being mere children and not necessarily altruistic, will use anything to get what they want. By the time he is six years old, a kid will realize that making Mom feel guilty about dating will get her to buy him banana splits, a keeno ten-speed just like Jimmy's down the street, and his very own hot tub. And if he really plays his cards right, he can even get her to take him to see two Disney movies *in a row.*

He'll often get away with this. But whenever you catch him at it, object fiercely. Say something like "Don't try that stuff on me, kid. Just because you're the most deprived kid on earth doesn't mean you don't have to do your homework. And no, I am not buying you a Harley-Davidson, you are only eight years old. Now hop to that homework."

A surefire way to alleviate guilt is to hire a good baby-sitter. A good baby-sitter is not a foul-tempered elderly person who speaks only German. A good baby-sitter is not a teenager who giggles on the phone all night. A good baby-sitter is not a convicted felon.

A good baby-sitter is someone you despise because your kid likes him better than you. A good baby-sitter has an endless passion for cataloguing baseball cards and Barbie Doll outfits. A good baby-sitter thinks it's a neat idea to phone drugstores and ask if they have Prince Albert in a can and if so will they please let him out. A good baby-sitter knows exactly who Luke Skywalker is, and is well versed on the latest developments of "General Hospital."

An even better baby-sitter is the parent of one of your kid's best friends who is deranged enough to actually let your child stay overnight, even though she will force you to reciprocate. You should scour the earth for this person, although ideally she will live on your block.

This way, when you bring someone home to spend the night, you can giggle and moan all you want, and no one will have to wrap a sheet around himself before venturing to the bathroom.

HOW MUCH SHOULD CHILDREN KNOW ABOUT YOUR SEX LIFE?

As little as you can get away with telling them. It's none of their business, and they're too young to know about it anyway.

Do not, on any account, get carried away in bed and start screaming if there is a child sleeping close by. Even if the kid was weaned on loud rock music, he could still wake up and think someone is hurting you.

Try to keep stray men out of your child's realm completely. When indulging in a vague, fleeting affair, do it when the kid is away from home. It can be emotionally scarring for a child to repeatedly wake up to find that there is a strange man wearing Mommy's frilly pink bathrobe in the kitchen. And that this mean man has just finished all the Froot Loops, and is he his new daddy or what?

When a meaningful man comes into your life, the kid will have to meet him. Keep the introductions simple. "Kid, this is Roger. Roger, this is the kid" will suffice. Try not to add "and I'm sure that the two of you will become very, very good friends."

And no "Uncle" stuff. The mother who says, "This is your Uncle Roger, darling," will soon have a wise-ass for a child.

The first time Roger spends the night, make it a jolly occasion. Do not loll around naked in bed until midafternoon, no matter how much you're dying for one more quickie.

Instead, just this once, be a good Brady Bunch kind of mom. Get up early, put on some dumb, demure housecoat, and go make pancakes. Kids think TV shows are real life, and if he sees you comporting yourself like Florence Henderson he'll be vastly reassured.

Then the two of you can go wake up good old Roger by tickling him to death. Roger had better be a good sport. He should also be wearing pajama bottoms or something. One doesn't want to be too modern.

(When your child reaches puberty, he will be fully cognizant of exactly what's transpiring and become insufferable. At this point you'll have to get him his own apartment.)

Accidents will happen. If your kid happens to be spending the night down the street, he could suddenly decide to favor you with a surprise visit. This happened to me once.

"Who's that?" Rex asked nervously as we heard a key turning in the lock.

"Who's that?" said the kid as Rex tried to grin at him nonchalantly from under the covers.

I performed formal introductions, but as far as social situations go, this one fell sadly flat. None of us even had the presence of mind to discuss the weather.

But things worked out okay, as they usually do. Later that week, the three of us saw a movie together and Rex taught the kid all about papier-mâché, something I shall never forgive.

As long as you love him, a kid can cope with all sorts of situations. Always remember that he will be leaving home one day to have a sex life of his own.

PSYCHOLOGICAL WEIRDNESS

The moment you bring a new fellow into your life, your child can get strange at a moment's notice, since it is a famous fact that children of divorced parents blame themselves for their parents' breakup. "If I were a better little tyke," the kid muses, "Mommy and Daddy would still be together. It was probably me spilling the milk all over the back seat of the car that did it."

So the kid appoints himself matchmaker. He tells Daddy how Mommy has some nice new nail polish now. He tells Mommy that Daddy just bought a terrific new drill, and why doesn't she call him and have him put up her bookshelves?

When Mom finds a new boyfriend, the kid tries his damndest to get rid of the interloper, who could ruin all his plans. He will spill ink on Mommy's new dress. He will develop appendicitis. He will ask Mommy's boyfriend how come he has such a stupid nose. He will douse the house with perfume so that it smells like a Mexican bordello. He will remember important homework just as Mommy is walking out the door.

I know a five-year-old girl who bursts into tears and demands her daddy whenever her mother's date appears at the door.

I know another little girl, an older and savvier one, who simply adores discussing her mother's cellulite with every new prospect on her mother's horizon.

It does not help to bribe the kid, although we all do it. ("Be good tonight when Jim comes over, Bobby darling, and Mommy will take you to the Bahamas.") Then we try manipulation. ("If you're not a good boy tonight, Mommy will get miserable and cry and cry.") Finally, in desperation, we threaten. ("Okay, kid, if you're not quiet tonight when Jim gets here, I'll cut off each and every one of your fingers.")

None of these methods works. But honesty, a novel approach, sometimes does the trick. You sit your kid down and say, "Look here, sweetums, your Dad and I are never going to get back together.

It had nothing to do with you when we split up, and nothing you can do or say will make us love each other again. So lighten up."

AND BOYFRIEND MAKES THREE

By far the worst peril of single motherhood is suddenly acquiring another child, and not of the infant variety. I've met many a hairy-chested male who immediately regresses to two-year-old status the minute he sees me tie my son's shoes.

"Well," the hairy-chested male muses, "she's already tying one set of sneakers, certainly one more won't make a difference. And what the hell, she can always throw one more lamb chop in the pan."

And then, when it turns out I can't throw *any* lamb chops in the pan, the hairy-chested man sulks. He refuses to understand why I won't mother him, too.

There is only one way to deal with a man like this:

Shout, cry, throw crockery and generally act like a two-year-old yourself. If he can cope with this, keep him around. He may well be the man for you, since a large part of any intimate relationship is taking turns being Mommy and Daddy. But it's no fun when it's all one-sided.

SELF-PITY AND THE SINGLE PARENT

You must not be sad when you meet fellows who don't want you because you have children. Such guys are not even worth a thought.

And if you decide to become all bitter and melancholy and full of a terrible sympathy for yourself, cut it out.

You have a kid, don't you? Kids are great stuff. They tell you your toenails are pretty just when you've convinced yourself you're the ugliest blimp on earth. They'll play Monopoly with you and you can usually beat them. They like it when it snows outside. They'll often share their teddy bears. They love you.

10

Sticky Situations

For the betterment of this chapter we have called in the famed Viennese psychiatrist Dr. Eva Rosa Anna von Sex Tips, who has graciously consented to bestow upon us her valuable perceptions and irrefutable logic. Dr. von Sex Tips' specialty is Sticky Situations in the modern female's life. I have assembled before her a panoply of the most commonly confronted situations of the sticky variety. Let's see how the old prune handles them.

DEAR DR. SEX TIPS:

There is this terrible twerp in love with me. Well, he's not really terrible, he's actually kind of sweet, but he's got this squeaky voice and weighs in at about 110, and I am particularly fond of your more beefy, basso-voiced male.

I do not want to offend this little twerp, since he works at the corner store and I don't want to have to travel four extra blocks to get my cigarettes. How can I let him down easy?

C.J.

DEAR C.J.:

First of all, my dear young woman, one must refrain from this vulgar and judgmental terminology. One girl's twerp is another girl's dreamboat, and I happen to know that you yourself are partial to cowboys with a pronounced gut and profuse facial hair—a type to which more than a few negative adjectives could apply.

However—on the rejection tactics. You are correct in assuming that saying "Fuck off, you minuscule wart, I hate your face" is not practical, not kind.

You have several more efficacious choices:

1. Plead insanity. Tell him you've enjoyed these lunches with him enormously but that your shrink, whom you visit six times a week, thinks that they aren't good for you, since you often become overexcited and start thinking you're a teapot again.

You think he's a wonderful guy, and you hate to give him up, but you're simply too mentally ill. Can he possibly forgive you and understand? Would he like to come to your weaving party at the clinic? Doesn't he think it kind of funny how flies talk in such flawless Serbo-Croatian?

If you're not sure he's fully convinced, phone him regularly at three in the morning and keep asking him why so many iguanas keep flying in the window.

2. Say your heart is no longer your own. Tell him that if it weren't for Moose, your six-foot-four All-American tackle boyfriend, you'd be happy to accept his extremely flattering advances.

3. Claim irreversible heartbreak. Yes, you appreciate his warmth, his affection. He is, in fact, aces with you. But doesn't he know that your heart was smashed to bits recently? That you never want to get involved with anyone, anytime, anywhere? No, no, you're sorry, but you won't reconsider—you know your own heart, and it's broken. You'll always think of him fondly, but you realize he's beginning to think too warmly of one whose heart is ashes. Best to cut it off right now, for everyone's sake.

4. You can't help yourself, you happen to be a lesbian. Be careful about using this one, since many a little twerp, in an effort to salvage a battered ego, will publicly call a girl a lousy diesel-dyke just to get back at her. There's not

a thing wrong with being a diesel-dyke, but it could become a bit disheartening when you go to a party and only women come on to you.

5. Try the truth. Say, "Herb, I've been thinking. You're a very jolly guy, a veritable prince. But something's missing. I guess it's that I like big, hair-infested cowboys. My friends will probably think I'm crazy to pass you up, but pass you up I must."

Many fellows will be too conceited to believe you, but it's worth a shot.

If all else fails, try THE FINAL SOLUTION:

Call him three, four, even five times a day to see how he is. Tell him you're dying to meet his mother. Perhaps you two and your respective mothers could get together for a nice rubber of bridge. And what kind of china pattern does he like? Does he believe in short engagements? Is he sure he really likes you? How much? Is he sure? If he likes you so much, why didn't he call you last night? Well, why didn't he keep trying? What does he have planned for New Year's Eve? How about the one after that? How many children does he want? Has he picked out any names yet? How about Jason and Jennifer? And Heather and Noah?

Any reasonable man will respond to this treatment by doing a creditable impersonation of a bat out of hell.

DEAR DR. SEX TIPS:

Now I've really done it.

There I was, minding my own business, when my best friend's boyfriend professed his unswerving lust and admiration for me.

You could have knocked me over with a feather. I was horrified yet pleased, indignant yet flattered. I started having an affair with him.

Then one day Fred (not his real name) found out that Ginger (not her real name) was, irony of ironies, cheating on *him*.

Well, Fred freaked. Went off his head completely.

Next thing I knew, he had told Ginger of our affair just to get back at her.

Whether or not Ginger feels guilty about her own actions is moot. All I know is, about a month ago she tried to run me down with her car. When I phone her, she hangs up. She hates me.

I don't want her to hate me. I've stopped seeing Fred now, that wimp in wolf's clothing, and I want my best friend back. How can I get her to forgive me?

CLAUDETTE

DEAR CLAUDETTE:

This is what comes of modern ways. Everyone does everything they want to, and then they get surprised and bewildered when someone tries to run them over in speeding automobiles.

Where are rules? Where is decorum?

Rule #1: Do not fuck around with your best friend's lover. It is simply not done. Think of your best friend's lover as a eunuch or, better yet, someone with no penis at all. This is not only sisterly, it is also the best way to look out for old number one.

When a girl gets herself entangled with a couple, she, most assuredly, is the one who will get hurt. Even if Fred were to leave Ginger for you, you'd still be out a best friend. But he probably won't leave her for you, and you probably don't even want him to. So where does the whole situation leave you? It leaves you as a pivotal character in someone else's soap opera, that's where it leaves you.

Rule #2: Never let a man get away with telling.

Fred, who is either an imbecile or an incredibly nasty son of a bitch, should be boiled in oil without further ado. By sleeping with you and then trumpeting it from the rooftops, he has forfeited his right to humanistic treatment. He has decided that you are a dispensable commodity, and massive retaliation is in order. Let it be known around town that he wears fishnet underwear and breeds miniature Chihuahuas. Bribe doormen to sneer at him. Throw banana skins in his path. Tell everyone the truth about him.

Re Ginger: Leave her alone for a while, she won't want to see your face and you can't blame her. Then, when you figure her ire has cooled, send her a telegram:

GINGER I MISS YOU AND MUST TALK TO YOU STOP IF YOU REFUSE TO SEE ME I WILL HAVE 20 PIZZAS DELIVERED TO YOUR HOUSE STOP EVERY NIGHT STOP THEN WHAT? STOP LOVE CLAUDETTE.

DEAR DR. SEX TIPS:

I don't know what to do. I'm thinking maybe I should kill myself. Or maybe I should kill him. I know I want to kill somebody. I also want to die. But possibly I should begin at the beginning.

I've been going out with Billy for eight months. He always told me he could never look at another woman.

But he can, and did. I was at a nightclub last week, when all of a sudden who should I see but Billy, sitting in a little secluded booth with a blonde. I was shocked, but convinced myself she was probably just a cousin from Peoria who liked dresses cut to the navel. But then, to my utter horror, I watched Billy take this tart in his arms and begin sticking his tongue down her throat.

Well.

I was traumatized and paralyzed, but eventually my legs came to and I ran sobbing out of the club.

Billy has been calling me every day. I keep hanging up on him. I never want to see him again. And yet, I still love him. That's why I want to die.

WANDA

DEAR WANDA:

You first must realize that you have two (2) very separate problems here: a cheating man, and unexpressed anger. It is the anger that's making you want to die.

The thing is, you blew it. There you were, all the evidence at your fingertips, but instead of taking command of the situation, you ran away. Not bright.

The proper procedure in this situation is to march up to the offending table and overturn it, taking care that at least three drinks, a lighted candle, and a large vase of flowers fall into that two-timing Lothario's lap.

Or, if you prefer to remain a stranger to violence, an equally effective procedure is to approach the philanderer's table with a grim smile on one's lips, wait patiently until the philanderer's attention is drawn to one, utter a few well-chosen icy syllables along the lines of "Aha!" and then march away stonily.

When this creature phones again, do not hang up on him. Tell him, in no uncertain terms, what you saw and what you think of him. Do not whine, do not cry. Keep the voice cold, aloof, and distant. Whining and crying are an admission of weakness and almost an engraved invitation to more ill treatment. They will only induce guilt, when it would be much more to the point to induce fear.

If he dares to accuse you of jealousy, have a screaming fit. Jealousy is one of the few honorable emotions we have, and anyone who claims not to be jealous is either lying or severely brain-damaged.

"Of course I'm jealous, you swine!" you should shriek, "and don't you *dare* try to manipulate me into feeling guilty for my jealousy or I'll come after you with a rusty rake!"

If he tries to lie his way out of the situation or, even worse, maintains that he has done nothing wrong, get rid of him. If he seems genuinely contrite and promises to be a lot more faithful in the future, give him another chance.

DEAR DR. SEX TIPS:
I have been living with Nathan for three years. The first year was unmitigated bliss, heaven and paradise. I thought Nathan and God were interchangeable. And Nathan is sweet, smart, and witty and loves me within an inch of my life.

But I am bored. To distraction. I have taken to clipping coupons and having my hair done four times a week. I think if Nathan says, "Wanna watch Carson, or what?" one more time, I am going to attack him with a meat cleaver.

For a while I was afraid of leaving, afraid of being on my own, afraid there was something wrong with *me*, not him.

But there isn't. I'm fine, and I want out.

I just can't bring myself to tell Nathan. Shall I tell him while he's humming happily over his morning coffee and the inevitable slice of dry whole-wheat toast? Shall I tell him when he comes home from the gym at 7:30, asking, "What's to eat, sweets?" Shall I tell him after he takes the garbage out at 9:30?

Everything in our lives is so prosaic and ordinary, I simply can't see myself suddenly saying, "Nathan, I'm leaving you." What to do?

JENNIFER

DEAR JENNIFER:

There is no optimum time to break up with someone. No matter when you tell him, you're going to blow the whole day.

If I were you, I'd take "Wanna watch Carson, or what?" as my cue.

"No, Nathan," I'd say. "Let us not watch Carson tonight. Let us instead divide up our philodendron and figure out who's getting the Cuisinart."

If Nathan says, "Oh, thank God, I've been trying to bring this up for months, but just didn't have the nerve to tell you," you're home free. But chances are he won't.

Chances are he'll threaten suicide, in which case you'll have to tap your gentlest, kindest resources. Leaving a lover is a stunning, crippling blow, and we're lucky that no one can arrest us for assault and battery.

But you must be firm. If Nathan wants to keep you, he'll try every trick in the book. He'll lock himself in the bathroom and refuse to come out. He'll lock you in the bathroom. He'll have his mother, father, siblings, and assorted cousins visit you and cry. He'll call your clergyman. He'll wet the bed. He'll stay out drinking all night and pass out in your front yard at 10 A.M. He'll take up heroin and hookers. He'll invent new sex techniques. He will continually remind you of nostalgic moments. He'll play "Stand By Your Man" on a repeating tape loop.

But you will have none of it. Oh, you'll be nice, all right, but you'll brook no nonsense. "Yes, Nathan dear," you'll say, "I remember quite well that time that I got drunk and put the lampshade on my head and you carried me all the way home in a blinding snowstorm, but I'm still leaving you. It's necessary for my emotional growth."

Lay the "emotional growth" business on thick. You don't want to place the blame on him. If you were leaving him because he is a two-timing, lying, cheating, mean, nasty, and thoroughly rotten brute, you'd have every right to broadcast it internationally. But Nathan isn't a brute, he's just tedious. So you simply must talk a lot of rot about your own lack of maturity and need for time alone, not to mention space.

He may not believe this, but at least he'll have something to tell the fellows at the gym, and this is of paramount importance. Fellows always need something to tell the other fellows at the gym. This way he can say, "Yeah, Jennifer says she needs some more space. *Space.* Go figure women." And all the fellows at the gym can then nod sagely about the futility of figuring women and then coax Nathan into a rousing game of squash to get his mind off you.

As soon as you've dropped your bombshell, move out. The place will turn into a veritable morgue until you do, and the recriminations will keep on coming. If you can't pack up all your belongings immediately, make sure to get your true valuables out pronto, since hell hath no fury like a man scorned. You could return to pick up your valuable collection of 45s only to find that Nathan has melted them.

As soon as you're out, you'll probably start having second thoughts. After about two weeks, the vision of Nathan (dear sweet old Nathan!) taking out the garbage will conjure up a misty feeling inside of you. You'll begin to wonder what you could have been thinking, giving up so capital a fellow. And then when you're walking down the street one day and see dear sweet Nathan with a curvy brunette, you'll know you've been a fool.

DEAR DR. SEX TIPS:
Is it ever a good idea to have an affair with a married man?

I have to admit I'm contemplating it heavily. In fact, I think about it all the time. Well, if the truth were to be known, I'm actually doing it.

Mario isn't your typical married guy. He doesn't try to tell me his wife doesn't understand him. He doesn't take me to sleazy motels. He doesn't get drunk on martinis and then sob and try to show me pictures of his children. He doesn't have his secretary send me flowers.

Mario is honest, forthright, extremely sexy, politically correct, sensitive, intelligent, and rich. And married. Oh, God, what am I doing? I mean, what can I *really* expect in this day and age?

What if he leaves his wife for me? What if he doesn't leave his wife for me?

SARAH

DEAR SARAH:
There are times when I feel (for even Dr. Sex Tips has feelings) that married men, as far as single women are concerned, are the scourge of the earth, the black plague and the eternal nemesis all rolled into one. That they are a rampantly out-of-control fungus which must be stopped before they put an end to human life as we know it.

At other times, in a more mellow mood, I simply feel they are minor disturbances, small crawly things that must be stamped on and squashed.

Here's why:

The first thing a married man will do, often within seven minutes of meeting you, is confess his love for you. His eyes will go all gooey and contrite—at this stage of the game he knows that only the wounded-animal approach will cut any ice—and he will start sending you long-stemmed roses and icy bottles of Louis Roederer champagne. If he's a smart married man, he won't even mention his wife and how she doesn't understand him—such a worn-out cliché at this juncture could prove disastrous. But he *will* suggest running off to Paris and touch heavily on the theme of never having met anyone quite like you before. He will wax profound upon your beauty, speak unceasingly of his uncontrollable lust for you, wonder wistfully what kind of children you two would produce, and propose to put a down payment on adjacent burial plots.

Very intense very quickly, your married man. It seems too good to be true, too romantic to be real. Even the most sensible of girls can be swept off her feet and start daydreaming about torrid scenes in airports.

And, of course, it *is* too good to be true. The intensity that a married man feels (and he really does feel it, he's not lying) could never exist in a member of the species who is single. Your married man can get as intense as he wants to, because he is safe. There, lurking quietly in the background, is his wife.

What is a wife? I hear you ask. She's not as pretty as me. She's older than me. She wears polyester. She's got a frumpy hairdo. What does she have that I don't have?

She's got her husband, that's what she has. The real, true fellow, the one who wakes up in the morning and complains that all his shirts are blue and he hates blue shirts. The one who dips his french fries in his coffee. The one who snarls if his soft-boiled egg is too runny.

A wife is the married man's safety net. With you he can be a dashing, moody, romantic and demanding lover. A paragon of sensitivity, vulnerable to a fault. Because he doesn't *need* you—he's got his security blanket waiting for him at home, keeping the teapot warmed. He has nothing to lose, he's playing the game with a stacked deck, and you have no aces.

You may not care. "Let him have his cake and eat it too," you may think. But there is another problem to contend with:

The enforced *passivity*.

You can't call a married man whenever you want to. If, at three o'clock in the morning, a huge water bug decides to set up light housekeeping on your living-room floor, you can never get a married man to rush right over with a machine gun. If you suddenly realize that you can't see the movie on Thursday at three as planned, you can't ring him up and change it to Tuesday at four.

You tend to wait around a lot. Even worse, things must be done at his convenience. "When can you get away?" you'll find yourself asking, as well as "Oh, you can't make it? Well, I suppose beef Wellington keeps pretty well in the freezer."

This sort of passivity tends to put a girl in a foul temper. You'll begin by resenting his wife, which will then make you irritated with yourself for resenting his wife when it's *his* goddamned fault. And then you'll become even more annoyed as you realize that it really isn't his fault, that nobody tied you up and forced you to have an affair with him.

Pretty soon every train of thought will arrive at the conclusion that you are an indefatigable louse, moron, and masochist. You'll start staring moodily into space and contemplating runaway trips to the Yucatán, where, you hear, they don't even *have* married men. You'll start thinking of yourself as some kind of sordid "other woman" and forget what a terrific pool player you are and how on numerous occasions you have been all that is wonderful to your querulous maiden aunt.

But the absolute worst thing about having an affair with a married man is that you must always be prepared for him to leave his wife for you and ruin everything.

When a man leaves his wife for you, he turns into a different person, a person you will find only vaguely recognizable.

Gone will be your intense, excruciatingly romantic lover. The flowers, whispered endearments, and passionate lovemaking will inevitably give way to whining about blue shirts and snarling at the sight of imperfectly cooked eggs.

No one is more insecure and unbalanced than a man who has just left his wife. He is a frightened man, a nervous man, a clinging man. And he will look to you to be his rock. Every time he wonders if he's made some awful mistake, he'll phone you up to make sure you really love him as much as you said you did yesterday.

You may find this somewhat endearing at first, but eventually the fear of suffocation will cause you to run screaming into the night.

And then where will you be?

The only even minimally suitable time to get involved with a married man is when you don't want to be immersed in anything heavy but still crave a bit of affection and intimacy.

I myself did this once, although I still found myself moaning and complaining about how stupid I was being One day my married paramour got a trifle annoyed with me and put down the pocket Space Invaders game and said, "Look, Eva Rosa Anna, you don't have anything else going on at the moment, do you?"

"Well, no."

"Then could you please shut up? You can just stick with me until something better comes along. I may be married to someone else, but at least I love you."

"Hah," I said.

DEAR DR. SEX TIPS:

I'm in love with a gay man.

At least, he's mainly gay, although I know for sure he's had two affairs with women.

But for the last several years he's confined his sexual activities to men. And yet, I think he's in love with me too. Whenever we're together, he never stops staring at me. He holds my hand, will often lean over and kiss me, and gets jealous when he sees me with other men. And I mean *really* jealous—screaming, ranting, sulking jealous.

I think about Tim night after night. All the time. We've never been to bed together, but he's always hinting he wants to. I think he's afraid. How can I encourage him?

CHRIS

DEAR CHRIS:

One must never fall in love with a gay man until *after* one has slept with him.

I have no doubt whatsoever that he is in love with you. Gay men often fall in love with women. Probably his dreams are riddled with visions of you running in gauzy dresses through fields of wildflowers. But will he come across?

The gay man–straight woman motif is famous. He loves her for her sensitivity, she loves him for his sensitivity. They laugh at the same '30s musicals. They both hate everything aqua. They fall in love. Often they end up sleeping together.

Often the sleeping together comes about when the woman, eager to get on with the main event, contrives to lose her keys at some nightclub at 3 A.M.

"Well, why not sleep over?" the gay man asks. The girl agrees. They go to his apartment. He whips them up a light snack—veal *aux champignons*, nothing fancy. They giggle together over his Zsa Zsa Gabor scrapbook, exclaim together over his collection of Art Deco saltshakers. They throw the I Ching.

Then it's time for bed. He strips down to his underwear and crawls between the sheets. The girl demurely does the same. He puts his arm around her. She snuggles close. He strokes her hair. She caresses his bicep. He falls asleep.

One of my patients was in love with a gay man for years. She spoke of the ugly scenes that ensued when she decided she wasn't having any more of the falling asleep business.

"Trying to get a gay man to have sex with you," she says, "is not a pretty picture.

"And the worst part is that as much as they love you, the fact that they can't or won't get it up is a terrible rejection. They don't necessarily mean to be cruel, but they are. At least the seductive ones are. The ones who lead you to believe."

So leave it. Put him firmly from your mind. If he starts chasing you around a bed and ripping your clothes off in a frenzy, you may then reconsider.

DEAR DR. SEX TIPS:

Every time a person turns around, someone is telling her not to get involved with someone she works with.

Is this really true? I live in a very large city, and the only men I meet are the guys I work with. I guess I could go to singles bars, but the idea doesn't appeal.

And now I find myself growing attracted to my boss. Every day and in every way we are becoming closer and closer. I know that, with just a little encouragement from me, we could have a romance in a minute.

Should I give him that crucial encouragement?

ETHEL

DEAR ETHEL:

It all comes down to the single, pivotal question—can you afford to lose your job?

Do you have an aging mother and three spinster aunts to support? Is this the job of your dreams, leading to certain fame, fortune, and inner peace? Are you on parole?

If so, give the boss a miss. When it comes to sex versus survival, one must regrettably opt for survival.

But if this job is not of the essence, what the hell, have a go—although it is better to carry on with one who doesn't have the power to fire you. Try someone in accounting or something. Someone who can help you figure out your expense forms.

And do not listen when busybodies tell you not to get involved with men at work. What do they know?

If you were in a small town, it would be different, be-

118 · *Sex Tips for Girls*

cause you'd know everybody. But in a big city, work is the closest thing you have to a community. So what if you break up and still have to look at him every time you pass the water cooler? In a small town, you'd probably see him every time you went to J.C. Penney for socks.

11

Sex Tips # 3—
How to Be Good in Bed

Although there is not a thing wrong with knowing every sex trick ever perpetrated in the history of womanhood, there are, in fact, only two (2) essentials to being a terrific lover: (1) manners, and (2) enthusiasm.

MANNERS

People with their clothes off tend to take things rather personally. Therefore, although there is a certain informality inherent in being naked, one must be even more strict with one's social graces. The Golden Rule, for example (which, in case it's slipped your mind, requires doing unto others as you would have them do unto you), should be closely observed. Be polite, be pleasant. It is not polite to

—laugh and point at the penile member
—break into prolonged, spasmodic sobbing
—say that your husband did it exactly the same way
—discuss running sores
—imitate Joan Rivers
—start snoring while one's partner's head is between one's legs
—ask if it's in yet.

Feel free to do any of the above if you want to sever relations with a man, since any one of them will cause him to disappear in no time. Otherwise, make tact your byword.

ENTHUSIASM

Do not keep your appreciation of sexual pleasures to yourself. I have a friend, I can't remember her name, who was once told by her lover that she was simply magnificent in bed.

"I am?" this friend said coyly. "Oh, no, I'm not really so special, am I? Really? No kidding? Why?"

"Because you really love to be fucked," her partner told her.

Think about it. Nothing arouses us so much as a man who seems to be hovering on the brink of insanity with sexual desire. If, in word or gesture, a man tells us something like "If I don't fuck you in the next six seconds I'll throw myself out the window," we tend to like this man an awful lot, and realize that we have here a man with excellent taste.

"So how," I asked my friend, "do you manifest this appreciation?"

"Oh, I dunno," she said casually. "I moan, I yell, I wriggle around a lot, I have been known to bite on occasion, I arch my pelvis eagerly, I smile, I plead and beg for more. . . ."

Plead and beg?

"Sure. Bed is one place where you're allowed to be greedy. So I tell him not to stop or I'll die. Stuff like that. And, I think this is probably important, I make it pretty goddamned clear to him that I don't do this sort of stuff with just anybody."

You don't?

"I don't. I only yell and moan and plead and beg with him, because he's the greatest lover in the world and I want to make sure he knows it."

"What's his phone number?" I asked.

Nonetheless, there are a few skills that it behooves a girl to master.

HOW TO PERFORM ORAL SEX

—Take the penis into your mouth and suck on it.

HOW TO PERFORM GOOD ORAL SEX

One must, first and foremost, understand the psychology of the penis.

Although the penis, when well on the road to climax, is strong, stalwart, singleminded, and ruthless, a penis in the first stages of erection is a sensitive little plant. You must be gentle and nurturing, coddle it until it grows big and strong.

(a) Start out by licking it affectionately. The head of the penis, when licked in a sort of swirly motion, will feel extremely cheerful.

(b) After you've paid sufficient attention to the head, you'll find that there is a ridge that runs straight down the underside of the penis that will simply be clamoring for equal time. When the pressure of the tongue is exerted on this ridge, the penis will start to throb with anticipation and the man owning the penis will gibber incoherently and offer you emerald earrings if only you don't stop.

(c) Stop at once. Take as much of the penis as you can get into your mouth. It will wonder why it didn't think of that itself. Suck gently, as if on a particularly captivating lollypop.

The penis should be fully erect by now. If it's not, run through (a), (b), and (c) again.

(d) When it is sufficiently rocklike in aspect, begin sucking in earnest. Your average penis, unlike your average clitoris, craves a good amount of pressure. It gets irritated with hesitant, ethereal gestures. So suck as hard as you want. If the penile substance is too large to fit comfortably in your mouth (something to be devoutly hoped), feel free to use your hand as a complementary force. The penis will be pleased. It will feel pampered, with its head in your mouth and its shaft being lovingly manipulated by your hand.

(e) Let your passion take itself anywhere it wants to, and be sure to let your hands roam into the outlying erogenous areas, but refrain from introducing your teeth into the proceedings. A man becomes suddenly wary when he feels teeth nibbling on his pride and joy. He immediately wonders whether you're the sort of girl who gets carried away in the nibbling department. These sort of qualms dramatically dampen ardor. So leave off even the most benign toothplay unless requested to do so in writing.

(f) The testicles (often known as balls, nuts, and family jewels) enjoy a little licking and fondling also, and become downright surly if they don't get any. Be gentle with them.

(g) You have now come to a crossroads. You must stop and ask yourself, "Am I merely giving the best blow job in creation or do I want to escalate to bigger and better things?" Or, even more simply, "Do I want this man to come in my mouth?"

If you're just dabbling and teasing, you won't want to get too rhythmical, and you'll want to keep the pace less than fervid. Something about hard, rhythmic, escalating sucking makes a penis go completely off its onion, and before it knows where it is, it has exploded.

So you want to tactfully draw away before the point of no return. The point of no return is when the penis seems to swell to about twice the size it was just seconds before and grows more insistent than may be considered seemly, while the testicles turn all small and hard and wrinkled. If this happens, prepare yourself to swallow.

HOW TO SWALLOW

Some girls simply revel in swallowing sperm, some can take it or leave it, and some get distinctly edgy at the whole idea. They're afraid they might throw up.

This is not a completely unfounded fear. You've probably noticed that if you shove a finger down your throat, you gag. Girls have been known to do this sort of thing on purpose after consuming an entire German chocolate cake with a side of banana mousse. The penis, if given its head, will act much like that finger, thrusting down the throat for all it's worth.

You must show it who's boss. When the penis tries to gain another inch of territory, stop it in its tracks with a decisive flex of the jaw muscles. Then deploy your tongue to man the barricades.

When the famous gush finally comes, let it. Don't try to swallow immediately, it's best to take stock of the situation first. Let it sit in your mouth for a moment and you'll realize it's not quite the imperial quart you had first imagined, but instead a highly manageable, slightly bitter-tasting teaspoonful. And if you do not focus overmuch on the vision of tiny tadpolelike spermatozoa wriggling about, but instead pretend you've got a mouthful of some sort of exotic aspic, the whole thing will go down most easily. Practice by eating oysters.

Some girls spit sperm out, but this is not considered sporting. And your partner will become despondent if you turn green, cross your eyes, and start dribbling into the corner of the sheet.

DEEP THROATING

Deep throating does not exist. It is a mythical practice allegedly perpetrated by pornographic film stars.

Like everything, it's done with mirrors. When the pornographic film director yells "Action!" the scantily clad actress positions herself underneath the male star's throbbing member; and cleverly slips this throbbing member behind her cheek. The hordes of greasy degenerates who watch these movies are completely bamboozled.

The only humans who can successfully perform deep throating are bona fide card carrying sword swallowers. Since most of these guys are tattooed and sweaty, your average heterosexual male will pass up the treat.

HOW TO GET A MAN TO PERFORM ORAL SEX

Some men love oral sex and will dive right for it with the slightest encouragement. If you find a man like this, treat him well. Feed him caviar and expensive brandy and don't let your girlfriends catch a glimpse of him.

But occasionally even the best of men will cavil at muff-diving. He will start glancing furtively at his watch and muttering about urgent appointments. One can understand this sort of man's feelings. And one can despise these feelings. It is every red-blooded girl's duty to put this sort of man straight. Pronto.

A few suggestions:

—Tell him you know for a fact that Burt Reynolds wouldn't be caught dead not giving a girl head.

—Gaze wistfully into the distance and say, "You *are* a pet, Harold, and I *am* devoted to you. But I'm afraid that no man can ever satisfy me. Ah, there was one time, very long ago, when I was thrilled and delighted beyond my wildest dreams (here's where you let a wistful smile play across your face). There was a man, you see, who put his head between my legs and well, ah, he *licked*. I was crazy with desire, Harold. I became a veritable animal. Ah, but (another wistful smile) I don't suppose I could ever hope to feel *quite* so passionate again."

—Tell him that you read somewhere, you think it was probably in *Forbes*, that the only men who make it into the top economic bracket are the ones who eat pussy on a regular basis.

—Next time you're walking down the street and spot a veritable Adonis, point to him and say, "Isn't Marcello over there amazing? You'd never guess that he's actually sixty-seven years old, would you? The doctors were baffled, but then they found that there is a certain youth-prolonging enzyme secreted by the vagina which, mysteriously enough, can be absorbed only by pressing the tongue directly on the clitoris. And the more you move the tongue in light, flicking motions, the more of this enzyme is absorbed into the bloodstream. Marcello's been lapping up this enzyme for years."

—Get into bed upside down.

—Tell him that any Pittsburgh Steeler not proficient in cunnilingus is not only ostracized but cut from the team.

If all else fails, you can always plead and beg.

HOW TO TALK ABOUT YOUR SEX NEEDS

1. Use tact.

When speaking with a friend, you, as the initiator of the conversation, must ask, "How are you?" and then wait for her to tell you. She, in her turn, will eventually ask, "And how are *you*?" Then, and only then, can you inform her that your hairdresser ran seriously amok and you're contemplating suicide.

Similarly, when you decide to inform your lover that he must stop treating your nipple as if it were chewing gum, it is best to first ask him how things are at his end. "Is there anything I could do that would make it better for you, pumpkin?" is a good introductory phrase. He may tell you, and you should take copious notes. And then he'll ask you how *you* are. Even if he doesn't, you may now feel free to tell him.

2. Use psychology.

Child psychology books are forever telling us not to be negative. Instead of saying, "Johnny, you must be subhuman if you can't read that word," we're supposed to say, "Johnny, you've done so wonderfully up to now, maybe if you just try a teensy bit harder . . ."

So try to remember that most of us are mentally still in swaddling clothes and will burst into tears and run away when confronted with overt criticism. "Stop treating my nipples like chewing gum, you abysmal wart hog" won't get you nearly as far as "I simply crave you when you suck on my elbows in that gentle way of yours. And my nipples, which are very sensitive, would like to be treated in exactly the same way."

3. Don't get cute.

There's something offputting about a girl saying, "Ooh, sweetie-poo, widdle Mona doesn't like it when you press so hard on her widdle love button."

4. If it can wait, let it.

When actually engaged in sex, one should try not to use words of more than one syllable. "Just put your tongue over here" is okay, as is "Why don't I get on top now?"

But if you have long, involved needs or critiques to relate, save them. The optimum time for these discussions is after the two of you have consumed your third margarita at a local bar and the bartender is out of earshot. Don't get carried away and make it five margaritas, or nobody will remember anything.

DOES SEXUAL BOREDOM EXIST?

Yes.

Incredible, yet true. There are times when even the most sex-crazed girl will turn to herself and say, "So what?"

HOW CAN WE CURE SEXUAL BOREDOM?

Expert opinion varies. Some say you must vary the time of day when you have sex. Others say you must vary the position. Still others suggest that you vary your personality. And plenty say that you must vary your costume.

The more discerning of you will notice a recurring theme in the abovementioned, a leitmotif. The more discerning of you will, in fact, jump headily to the conclusion that variety is the spice of sex. Jump ahead.

Vary the Time

Morning: As everyone knows, the best time of day to have sex is in the morning. The birds are chirping, the sun is streaming lazily through the window, and the man waking up next to you already has a hard on. No muss, no fuss.

Afternoon: Hordes of humans ignore the rampantly pleasurable experience of having sex in the afternoon.

Let us think upon the afternoon for a moment: a most tedious time period, usually devoted to picking up the dry cleaning.

Instead, why not fuck? It is extremely sluttish, wicked, and slothful to fuck in the afternoons, and therefore totally enjoyable. The ideal way to greet your lover on these occasions is in a see-through black floor-length negligee. Make sure you are also lying on a chaise eating bonbons and watching a soap opera. He, ideally, should come dressed as a delivery boy.

Evening: Unfortunately, too many people these days are indulging in sex in the evening, after they've gone to dinner involving some sort of nouvelle cuisine and seen the latest Steven Spielberg movie. This may be amusing in a kinky sort of way, but it often backfires. Nouvelle cuisine hopelessly confuses the stomach, which may protest far into the night. And Steven Spielberg movies, although charming, are prone to make one suddenly shout "E.T., phone home!" at inopportune moments.

Try this: When your date comes to pick you up for aforementioned dinner and movie, be not quite ready.

After you've found a vase for the roses he's brought and have given him a beer, decide it's about time you put on your garter belt. Make a big fuss of it. Prance around straightening seams and asking him if you have any runs.

"No, I don't think so," he'll say huskily.

"Oh, but they're wrinkling around my ankles," you can now complain, "I'll have to pull them up all over again."

"Could you come here a minute," he will at this point whisper hoarsely.

"No, I've got to figure out my stockings," say petulantly.

"I'll help you," he'll say. "*Please.*"

And there you'll be, missing your dinner reservation.

Night: How many of us have awakened in the night with nameless cravings?

If you happen to have a man beside you, do not shout "Fire!" in his ear and then say "Ha ha, only kidding, let's fuck." You could lose a valuable limb.

The proper procedure for waking someone for a quickie is this:

Gently stroke the sleeping man's penis and whisper barely audible obscenities in his ear. When he begins to stir, pretend you are fast asleep, rolling your pelvis a bit as if in the throes of an alluring dream. See if you can manage to position your bottom against his crotch, and roll your pelvis around a bit more. If he's the man we think he is, he will at this point make a sleepy grab for your breast, whereupon you should moan languidly and begin to burrow under the covers. This burrowing under the covers will give him ideas. Let him have them. When he gently guides your head even lower, act surprised.

VARY THE POSITION

You might want to try, just for an offbeat thrill, the missionary position. Although many trendsetters have dismissed the M.P. as passé, they're talking through their jaunty panama hats. The missionary position is terrific stuff: it allows for both passion and leverage, you can look into each other's eyes if you want to, and you can allow your legs an unrestrained freedom of expression. You can hook your heels around his ankles, you can twine your ankles around his neck, you can put your feet on his chest, you can wrap your legs around his waist. Each of these maneuvers is titillating and friendly.

Getting on top is dreadfully prosaic, but nothing beats it for the girl who likes to set her own pace. For an added thrill, get him to fondle your breasts. If he won't, fondle them yourself.

Sex while standing up can be amusing as long as you don't try to get too cute. Getting too cute means that you decide out of nowhere to throw your arms around his neck and legs around his waist so he has to carry you around, much the way Jack Nicholson seemed to be doing to Sally Struthers in *Five Easy Pieces*. A normal man can easily break both legs if you do this. You should try it only with a rookie linebacker whose knees haven't given out yet. Otherwise you should be backed up against a wall or he should be standing behind you.

There is a certain sexual position called "doggie-style," and I've never understood why. What I mean is, have you ever seen dogs doing it? Dull. Possibly a little panting, but absolutely no moaning or crooning, "Oh baby, oh baby." The female dog keeps her eyes open the whole time, wearing on her usually expressive face a world-weary expression more suitable for snubbing Brand X dog food.

When human girls do it doggie-style, they have a lot more fun, and here's why: They can't actually *see* their partner, and can pretend he's anyone. Benjamin Franklin, Napoleon, and Charles Dickens are particular favorites, or you can get really strange and not only pretend that he is Fidel Castro but also that you are Margaret Thatcher. The possibilities are endless.

VARY YOUR PERSONALITY

It is a famous theorem that, if a girl wants to be a sex goddess, she must be able to transform herself into a sultry wench, a blushing virgin, an untamed slut, an elegant courtesan, or a filthy whore at a moment's notice. Men, we are told, love this.

Men do not love this. In fact, there is nothing that shatters a man's nerves faster than not knowing, when he rings a woman's doorbell, whether he is to be confronted with Mata Hari or Pollyanna.

The world is sufficiently populated with schizophrenics. If a man wanted one, he could simply place an order at the nearest mental hospital.

VARY YOUR COSTUME

We, being modern and liberated and fully cognizant of women's sexual, intellectual, emotional, and economic oppression, can never for a moment cease our vigilance against the imperialistic male supremacist. We must never relax our guard against his chauvinistic sexual fantasies.

So don't even for an instant consider keeping the following hidden in the back of your closet:

—A see-through nurse's uniform complete with white seamed stockings and peaked cap.

—A cheerleader's costume, including large crepe-paper pom-poms and little red majorette boots.

—A little black French maid's outfit, involving a short black dress, frilly white apron, lace cap, feather duster, black-patent high heels, no panties, and fishnet stockings.

And if you do, don't tell anyone.

12

Inner Dieting

"Life is a banquet and most poor suckers are starving to death."

—AUNTIE MAME

If a woman is fat, or semi-fat, she probably falls into one of four categories:

1. *The Fearful Fat Person* (FFP)

According to the 2,000-year-old Man (a.k.a. Mel Brooks), fear is at the root of almost all everyday activities. Fear caused people to shake hands, dance, sing, get married, and was, back in caveman times, even the means of transportation ("An animal would growl and you would run two miles in a minute"). But Mel neglected to mention that fear is the major cause of fatness in America today. Fear has caused people by the hundreds of thousands to stop living and start eating.

When a FFP was growing up, she took the ridiculous adage "Better to be safe than sorry" and implanted it into her heart, where it grew and festered and turned her blood weak, her brain watery, and her stomach bloated. Instead of actually *living*, which entails too many petrifying risks, a FFP eats a jelly doughnut. Food is the only kind of adventure she permits herself, and it is not pleasant to observe the lengths she will go to avoid any bigger challenge than consuming pastrami on rye and a double chocolate malted on an empty stomach.

Principal characteristics of the FFP:

—She's taken out plenty of life insurance.

—She actually likes hors d'oeuvres and will, when arriving at a cocktail party, station herself next to the buffet table, where the constant consumption of chicken livers wrapped in bacon gives her a devil may care feeling and enables her to avoid talking to anyone.

—She hates her job, hates it, hates it, hates it. But she's afraid to leave because then she won't have the money for all those life-insurance premiums.

—When the coffee lady rings the bell at her office, the FFP goes running. She bites into a glutinous apple turnover and feels extremely secure, at one with the universe.

—She thinks it's fine to come home after work and have several martinis and a box of chocolates in front of the TV set.

—She reads self-help books and listens to her elders.

—She has sporadic fits of self-loathing that prompt her to go on crazy crash diets on which she is only allowed to eat pineapple. She doesn't understand why these never work.

—She and her friends often get together to discuss the meals they've had recently.

Many an FFP used to be a normal person, but a life trauma of some sort, often a stupidly painful love affair, has caused her to withdraw from the slings-and-arrows business.

Me, for example. When I was nineteen and 125 pounds, I fell in love with the most charming son of a bitch on earth. I was a rampant hippie then, living by my wits and waking up wherever I wanted to. Men were a pleasant diversion until I met this lethal man who broke my heart. I was devastated.

So devastated that within a year I had eschewed my jolly way of life, met and married a nice, safe, and sensible man, moved out to the suburbs and got fat.

I'm not talking a little chubby, I'm talking 162 pounds. I lived for devil's-food cookies. I ate them until I wanted to puke, but didn't. Actual life was too horror-prone for me, so the most exciting thing I did with my time was go to shopping malls and eat the free cheese samples.

Then one day I had a supreme fit because my husband didn't buy me two pounds of chocolates for Valentine's Day. I'll never forget myself. I was like Joan Crawford on angel dust.

"How *dare* you, you malevolent moron!" I shrieked.

"But there's a blizzard outside," he said reasonably. "You can't walk more than two feet without becoming snowblind."

"I don't care, I don't care, I *don't care!* I want my candy!"

Horrifyingly enough, I got my candy. But at about 4:30 that morning I awoke from a vivid nightmare in which I had a featured role as a pig in pink satin pajamas. I had a troughful of buttercreams but was forbidden to leave the sty. I woke in a cold sweat, wondering who I was and how I had got this way.

I tossed and turned and finally realized that unreconstructed pain had turned me into a rampant coward.

So I moved to London, got a job with a theater group, and started running around like a maniac again.

What with the fluctuating pound, you can't move to London every time you get fat. But everyone has the potential to change her life drastically and should keep doing so until she gets it right.

If you're a FFP, you should probably leave home. If you won't leave home, leave your job. If you won't leave your job, leave your husband. Somewhere, some way, somehow, you have to start taking risks again. You're going to die eventually anyway, at which point you'll be as safe as houses.

2. *The Angry Fat Person* (AFP)

The AFP never got enough breast milk as a baby, and her unconscious is still absolutely furious about it.

"Fuck everyone, I'll show them," the AFP thinks way down deep inside herself. "I'll eat as much as I want, whenever I want, whatever I want, and no one can stop me!" The fact that no one has tried to stop her for twenty years doesn't occur.

Since not getting enough to eat was the AFP's first angry experience, she translates any and all anger-provoking situations into a food-deprivation trauma. If she has a fight with her boss, she consumes a pound of pasta to get back at him.

She also feels that she must reward herself when she's been good, since none of those other bastards will. Sometimes she's so good she consumes an entire chocolate cake.

Distinguishing characteristics of the AFP:

—Instead of yelling at anyone, she eats.

—She's positive that her life is tougher than anyone else's.

—She's still not speaking to her mother.

—She trusts no one, and cannot refrain from hiding food in the most unlikely places. There are macaroons in her filing cabinet, jars of chocolate syrup in her underwear drawer, meringues in her medicine chest.

—She eats like a bird in public, then rushes home to hit the medicine chest.

—She spends a lot of time in bed—the combination of unexpressed anger and constant sugar overdose keeps her in a state of chronic clinical depression.

If you suspect you're an AFP, you have to practice expressing your fury instead of eating it away. Every time you have the urge for a cookie, take a hammer and smash the shit out of any pillows you happen to be around while you shout, "Take that, you bastard!" Cry and scream at every available opportunity. Lie down on the floor and kick your feet and flail your arms and hold your breath until you think you may be turning blue. You'll feel like a terrific fool but you'll start losing weight.

You may also want to equip yourself with a nice king-sized baby bottle to suck on at random moments. This will really tune up your jaw muscles, a great sexual asset. But leave the bottle at home before going to a job interview.

3. *The Man-hating Fat Person* (MHFP)

She's frightened of sex and men but won't admit it. So she gets fat, figuring that the rolls of flesh falling from her thighs will keep those terrifying male creatures at bay.

The MHFP's predominant characteristic is excessive bitterness. Some become radical feminists for all the wrong reasons. Then they stage huge fights with their sisters and retreat to the nearest delicatessen. Some become lesbians for all the wrong reasons and pick vicious fights with their lovers.

If you are a MHFP, you must delve deep into your psyche and try to figure out when it was that you first started despising men.

Was it when your father threw you out the window? When your cousin Joe took off all your clothes and locked you in the pantry? Then teach yourself, slowly but surely, to realize that all men will not throw you out the window or lock you in the pantry. Some of them will take you to the theater instead.

4. *The Bona Fide Fat Person* (BFP)

Some people are supposed to be fat and that's that. A bona fide fat person is completely content with her lot. You can recognize her by the following characteristics:

—She wouldn't give up asparagus with hollandaise or chocolate mousse for anyone or anything.

—She's a great dancer.

—She wears stylish, sometimes almost flamboyant, clothes and has no self-consciousness about her looks—although she will say, if someone should ask, that she won't wear dirndls because they make her look like a Volkswagen. She never wears frills or puffy sleeves because she knows that on a fat person they just look apologetic.

—She gets laid as often as any of us.

—Although she may have a sharp sense of humor, she won't make self-deprecating jokes.

—She likes to drink and is appalled at the idea of stopping.

—Her self-confidence verges on the arrogant.

—The idea of exercising fills her with horror and dread. Exercise, she believes, is fine for the lower classes, but walking to the corner to buy a newspaper is fine for the likes of her.

—Big is better than boring, she figures.

The interesting thing about the BFP is that people hardly ever notice. Most fat people walk around wearing a hangdog expression, awful clothes, and refuse to dance at parties. And since people are notoriously fond of feeling superior to anybody they can, an insecure fat person is a prime target for nasty jokes and malignant condescension. But a BFP has no notion, won't even tolerate the idea, that there's anything wrong with her, which makes it impossible for people to patronize her.

BFPs are rare and refreshing. The only problem they face is becoming too fat, which will kill them.

Do you recognize yourself in any of the above? All of the above?

Possibly not, and possibly, like 88 out of 100 women, you think you're fat just to give yourself trouble.

We all do it. We take a look at our waists, perfectly fine waists, and somehow they look as if they would be more at home on an elephant. We look at our upper arms and raise our eyes heavenward, wondering why God thought it was a fun idea to make them look like sausage links. Nobody, but nobody, is as fat as she thinks she is.

Here's how to tell if you're fat or simply letting your girlish high spirits go mental on you. Take a walk through your local shopping district. Make sure there are plenty of plate-glass windows in the vicinity. Stroll along, thinking of this and that, and then, when you're least expecting it, shoot a quick glance at a particularly shiny window. Look away quickly and form a mental picture of what you saw. Are there any blimps in that mental picture? If so, are any of the blimps wearing a green dress just like yours?

Another way to tell is to take the upper-arm pinch test. This entails taking the index finger and thumb, pinching the flab on your upper arm and then measuring it. If you can do this without bursting into tears or suffering a *petit mal*, you're not fat.

If you are, please read on.

HOW TO DIET

Most diets do not, I repeat, *do not*, work. Even fasting doesn't work, since you mainly lose water weight. The Stillman Diet involves ketones in your urine—something no girl really needs. Ditto the Atkins Diet. The Beverly Hills Diet is just silly, and if you stay on it for more than two days you'll start singing "My Way" and spend entirely too much time in the bathroom. The Scarsdale Diet isn't too bad, but it's not too good either, since its permanent results are flimsy at best. A lot of women I know swear by the Scarsdale Diet, and all of them are at least chubby. The Pritikin Diet is fine, although tedious.

I'm sorry to be such a bore, but if you want to lose weight you'll have to exercise. Not only does exercise burn up calories, but, even more important, when your body is composed of more muscle and less fat, your metabolism is more efficient and you can eat more and gain less.

Fat, like misery, loves company. Give your body fat a candy bar and it will embrace it happily, introduce it around to all the neighboring fat, and throw a housewarming party in your hips. Muscle, on the other hand, is snobbish. Introduce a candy bar to muscle and it will cut it dead. "My God, the awful riffraff that's being let into this body nowadays," muscle will murmur scathingly to the ill-bred Nestlé's Crunch as it turns it into pure energy and sends it on its way.

For exercise techniques, turn to Chapter Thirteen.

Once you start exercising, you'll be more in the mood to diet. It's funny how irritatingly wholesome your body can get if given the least bit of encouragement. Some people, after embarking on a program of exercise and diet control, have been known to give up smoking, drinking, and drugs. The mind boggles.

THE LOW PROFILE DIET

This is a good diet to start with, since it doesn't make its presence unduly felt. One usually knows it's time for the Low Profile Diet when, just as you're falling asleep one night, you get a visit from your guardian angel.

"Hsst, fatty!" your guardian angel will whisper in your ear.

"Are you talking to me?" you'll ask, unconsciously imitating Robert de Niro in *Taxi Driver*.

"Who else is there?" the angel will respond. "You haven't let a man see your body for *months*. Listen, sweetheart, I've been thinking. You've gotta take off some tonnage. You haven't been able to get into your great black jeans since last summer. How are you going to have a good time if you can't fit into your great black jeans?"

"You may have a point, you little devil."

"Angel, dollface. So listen, knock off the sweets for a bit, won't you? Not too much butter. No Eggs Benedict until further notice. Are you listening to me?"

No, you're not. You've fallen asleep. But in the morning you'll wake up all cheery and determined. You'll have a bit of grapefruit and toast for breakfast, possibly a spoonful or two of low-fat cottage cheese. You'll be delighted with your heroism.

About two hours later, you'll be flat on your back with hunger pangs. Visions of buttered and jammed croissants will dance into your head. Food, you'll think to yourself, is more important than sex, than getting into your great black jeans, than *anything*.

You have come to a crucial moment in your diet, and if you do the wrong thing, you're dead.

When hunger pangs strike, *you must eat*.

Have another piece of toast. Put a little butter on it this time. Have a glass of apple juice. Yes, this is all part of the Low Profile Diet, which is what makes it so wonderful.

When a girl goes on a traditional diet, she tries to convince her body that she hasn't been eating Oreo cookies and bacon sandwiches with alarming abandon. But her body knows better, since her stomach is accustomed to large amounts of food and her blood is addicted to heavy doses of sugar. If she tries to shrink her stomach in a day and go cold turkey on the sugar, she'll become suicidal.

Easy does it. For the first month of the Low Profile Diet, simply concentrate on eating whole-grained bread instead of croissants, eating fruit instead of pastry, and making sure you drink six to eight glasses of unsugared liquids a day. Dilute your fruit juice with water. Take your vitamins.

Of course you'll fuck up and eat seven brownies one fine afternoon. On a conventional diet, this is the moment you'd quit. "Well, I obviously blew it," you'd be saying to yourself in a self-pitying sort of way, helping yourself to an eighth brownie. "I may as well give up altogether."

Instead, just make these binges part of the diet. Don't deprive yourself unduly. But keep an image of yourself in those terrific black jeans plastered across your brain.

Eventually, in two weeks to a month, your stomach will have shrunk and your sugar cravings will have abated and you'll really get into it. This is when you can go into high gear, when not eating will be more satisfying than eating, when you become positively obsessed with how wonderful you're beginning to look.

Just don't get too crazy and decide to eat nothing. You might faint on the street.

And be careful about vomiting. Plenty of girls have been known to go into the bathroom after a particularly calorie-laden meal and stick their fingers down their throat. This is unsavory and also habit-forming. They have a name for this disease, bulimia. Turns out that once one gets started down this road, it's hard to stop. People have been known to consume 50,000 calories at one sitting, and then puke it all back up. Appalling.

Don't give up chocolate unless you're passionately in love and divinely happy. It seems that chocolate contains some sort of "happiness enzyme," which is produced by the body only when the body is having the best time ever. This enzyme makes you walk along the street whistling happy tunes and embracing random passersby. That's why you crave chocolate when you're depressed. Your body, as usual, knows what it's doing.

When you've lost enough weight to fit into your black jeans, you can stop dieting. If you've been exercising, you probably won't gain the weight back. But keep trying on the black jeans, just to make sure.

"But," I hear you say, "I want to lose ten pounds in the next two minutes. And I bet you've got a little something up your sleeve to help me do this. Out with it."

No I don't. I know nothing. I'm innocent.

"Oh no you're not," I hear you saying again. "You know something, we can tell. Your readers aren't imbeciles."

Well I don't actually *know* anything, but I have to admit that I was once at the public library reading Adelle Davis's *Let's Eat Right to Keep Fit*—just minding my own business, you understand—when suddenly, out of the middle of the book, fluttered a folded piece of grimy parchment.

"Oho," I said to myself, "what's this?" I unfolded the page to find closely scrawled, barely discernible handwriting. I read haltingly, and realized that I had come upon the most depraved diet plan I had ever laid eyes on.

I have no idea if it works. I wouldn't try it myself, God knows, and I certainly wouldn't recommend it to anyone. But here it is:

THE SEX & DRUGS & ROCK & ROLL DIET

For this diet to work, you must be in a properly delinquent frame of mind. To find out, take this quiz:

If you had your choice, would you rather

(a) Become the first female major-league pitcher?

(b) Have the man you love phone you and say he's got a gram of cocaine and some pretty new underwear for you and he'll be right over?

(c) Travel by yourself down a winding country road in the late spring in a small Maserati?

(d) Sing a duet with Mick Jagger in front of many screaming fans?

Well? If you're paralyzed with indecision, if every idea seems too appealing for words, you're ready for the Sex & Drugs & Rock & Roll Diet.

Follow these instructions to the letter. No substitutions.

1. Go out and buy the following things: a see-through negligee, a week's worth of supplies from a health-food store, a bottle of supervitamins, the kind of rock-and-roll records that make you jump around, twenty Quaaludes, and two grams of cocaine.

2. Look around for someone to have sex with. This is the tough part. The kind of person you want is a humorous, brilliant, eccentric, and passionate singer-songwriter with a cult following who never sleeps and burns himself out every chance he gets. You'll want him to go on the road often to give you recovery time. This guy may be hard to find, since the only living example of this species lives in a log cabin in Nashville. You may have to content yourself with anyone you're crazy or semi-crazy about. If you can't find anyone after two weeks, go get a cute guy from Houston or Fort Lauderdale, where they're all dying to get laid. Make sure you like him a lot.

You are now ready to begin.

Day One

Jump out of bed in the morning and immediately do:

2–4 lines of cocaine, well chopped.

1 cup yogurt, unsweetened.

Then go to a gym that specializes in weight training. None of those la-di-da health clubs with pools and saunas, they'll just make you boring and stupid. Work out and get it over with.

Do a little work. (If you have to go to an office, try not to talk to any fools while you're there, and every time you feel the urge for a jelly doughnut, go into the bathroom and do a fingernailful of cocaine.)

Finish work and find your sweetie. He's probably wandering

around the seedy side of town with strange lyrics running through his brain. Sneak your hand inside his trousers and he will immediately follow you home.

Before going to bed, eat as much health food as you can stand. Take a vitamin.

Try to have sex by no later than 6 P.M. This is really the start of your day.

Around midnight, get out of bed and either play your records and dance around or go out and dance around. Maybe take a long drive (pulling over to the side of the road for frequent sex) to another city and dance around there. Sing, too. Have a little cocaine. Take some Quaaludes and get really silly (optional). Whenever you have the urge to get drunk, take a Quaalude. Quaaludes straight won't make you nearly so obnoxious as Quaaludes with alcohol, a very bad and sometimes deadly combination. Do not, under any circumstances, drive when on Quaaludes. Even if you can drive perfectly when you're completely blotto on booze, the Quaaludes will make you drive straight into a tree. They can also give you a vile hangover.

Day Two
Same as day one.

In fact, follow this strict regimen for a week. You will lose ten pounds. At this point you must sleep for a day and a half or you'll die. Turn off your telephone.

After this first week, you will be completely attuned to your new way of life and can mix things up. Have sex before going to the gym if you feel like it. Skip the blow in the morning, or skip it at night. Or skip the blow altogether. It just makes you ignorant. Only go back to it when you feel the urge to eat cookies and watch television instead of donning your stockings and attacking your sweetheart.

And that's it. I can't imagine what the author of this diet could have been thinking. Everyone knows the drugs described therein are illegal and potentially dangerous.

Remember this: People who spend their time on the edge always look slender and bright-eyed.

13

Why Exercise?

"Why exercise?" the right-thinking girl rightly thinks to herself. "Why not just lie around in hammocks all day, sipping frequently from conveniently placed pitchers of margaritas, listening to the random play of crickets in hedges, smoking eight cigarettes at once and happily reading about the latest imposters at Blandings Castle?"

The R.T.G. has a point. Exercise, although a fine activity for the lower order of mammal who has to run fast in case something wants to eat it, may be totally unnecessary for R.T.G.s such as yourself. Just as long as you have the following credentials:

1. You are lean and sinewy and often mistaken for a gazelle.
2. Your body is a stranger to cellulite, ditto hanging flab.
3. Your upper arms can defy even the most intense scrutiny.
4. You simply never get headaches.
5. Or backaches.
6. You can dance for three hours straight with the partner of your choice.
7. Chocolate mousse means nothing to you.
8. You can pick up an electric typewriter (office model) and carry it jauntily for five or six blocks.
9. You can drink yourself into oblivion whenever you want to

and still spring out of bed every afternoon, eyes bright and shining, brain quick and jolly, ready to face whatever fresh horrors the day has in store.

10. You can spend several fast-and-furious hours of lovemaking without your masseter muscles giving up, or your pelvic girdle collapsing.

If the above credentials describe you to the point of being an actual self-portrait, you may stay in your hammock with equanimity. If not, pushups are in your future.

So throw your head back, grit your teeth, and go to it. Be brave. The only thing you have to fear is people pointing and laughing at you as you cower in your gym shorts, and to listen to them shriek with unbridled merriment while you attempt a single pushup, and fail.

If I can do it, so can you. I was (possibly still am) the prototypical wimp, the one who cried in gym class. Then one day my thighs threatened to secede from my body, and despair overcame fear. I started working out, and am now able to find my biceps. I arm-wrestle with twelve-year-olds and win.

WORKING OUT AT HOME

This is an attractive idea, but not a good one. It's true that one day you may find yourself overcome with energetic zeal and rush to the nearest sports shop where you'll buy $167.00 worth of weights, sweatbands, jump ropes, and how-to books, fully intending to wake up every morning and cavort about, but if your zeal lasts for more than three days you should be canonized. Working out alone is discouraging, especially if you get yourself one of those little books which tell you to turn to page 143 right after you've done exercise seven. One keeps losing one's place. One can't understand the pictures. One gets fretful. One decides to go back to bed and forget about it. One is right.

So ask around, find a good exercise class. A good class has a teacher who is cute (or at least witty), and who never tells you to go on a beansprout diet. A good class should have a number of students with excellent bodies to set an example, but there should also be a few other dodos to keep up your spirits.

Eventually you can go it alone, since exercising is addictive. Once your body gets used to regular workouts, it gets foul-tempered when deprived. Hard to believe, but there you are.

To become a muscular powerhouse-gladiator of a girl, your body needs three sorts of workouts.

AEROBICS

Contrary to popular cable TV-induced opinion, aerobics have absolutely nothing to do with squeezing your body into hideous shiny Spandex, grinning like a deranged orangutan, and doing cretinous dance steps to debauched disco music.

Aerobics are, in fact, the sorts of exercises that keep your heart pumping happily away, keep your lungs in good humor and your blood coursing merrily through your veins. They also keep you from gaining weight. No kidding. Aerobics three times a week can easily turn you into the sort of women to whom the Duchess of Windsor would have pointed to illustrate her theories. ("Don't look now," one can picture the Duchess saying to a nearby acquaintance, "but that woman coming toward us is the living illustration of my famous remark that you can never be too rich or too thin.")

Here's how aerobics work: Every single one of your muscles is riddled with glucose—simple sugar. As soon as you start jumping around, the sugar gets used up. Your muscles become bereft, they don't know where to turn. Eventually they hit on a solution and start plundering your fat cells. And presto! You're a beanpole!

Another truly heartening thing about aerobics is that they do something or other to your metabolic rate, I'm not sure what, but you can suddenly eat more without gaining weight.

Aerobic exercises include the following:

Running (not recommended—too '70s and involves frequenting reservoirs)

Bicycling

Swimming (highly recommended by Those Who Know)

Jumping rope

Intense sports like racquetball and squash (but not tennis)

Jumping around on a trampoline

Intense sexual activity

Imitating Mick Jagger

Imitating Mick Jagger is the most sophisticated form of aerobics. To do it properly, you must be very careful not to lapse into being Keith Richards. Keith, although often more compelling than Mick, is not aerobically sound, since he mainly just stumbles.

Also you must not imitate Mick when he is merely lying around watching TV and having a little snack. Instead, imitate him performing songs like "Shattered," "She's So Cold," "It's All Over Now," "Honky-Tonk Woman," and, of course, the ever-popular "Satisfaction." Eschew songs like "Wild Horses" and "Angie."

When you can perform eight to ten songs without passing out, consider yourself aerobically fit.

STRETCHING

Also called "flexibility training," stretching seems of minimal importance—just something you do when you wake up—until one day you notice a dancer take her ankle and put it nonchalantly behind her neck. Then, naturally, all the ramifications are manifest, and one understands why men are always fantasizing about dancers.

Stretching keeps the muscles fluid and elastic, and if you don't stretch before and after other types of exercising you'll be in serious trouble. Your entire body will seize up, much the way Peter Sellers' did in *Dr. Strangelove*. Stretching also keeps the muscles toned, firm, and cute. And just think of how interesting it could be to put your ankles behind your head while a man is on top of you.

WEIGHT TRAINING

Do not scurry back to your hammock in alarm—weight training can be fun. Well, okay, not actually *fun*, but mildly amusing. Weight training is nothing fancy, it just means making your muscles strong. However, you can probably never be a mass of bulges the way Arnold Schwarzenegger is, since most of us simply don't have the requisite amount of testosterone. Which, if you were to ask me, is a good thing, because along with bulging muscles, testosterone produces copious amounts of facial hair. Unless you want a job in a carnival sideshow, this will get you nowhere.

You can use any of those fancy machines or you can lift free weights.

But don't try lifting five-pound cans of tomatoes in your own home or you'll become profoundly despondent. You need real, heavy-duty weights.

To have the best time, every time you pick up a weight or push against the nautilus machine, simply pretend you are lifting a cheating lover or your snotnosed boss in preparation for throwing him/her down a long flight of stairs. Not only will this build up your strength, but you will develop the sunniest disposition in town.

CLASS ETIQUETTE

Since each of these programs initially requires classes, one must learn how to comport oneself.

First of all, make sure you arrive at class in dirty pink, stained white, or tattered gray leotards sporting plenty of holes and frequent rips. Leg warmers must be frayed. If you arrive all spanking fresh and clean, you will be shunned and forced to perform complicated arabesques in the hall.

Learn to breathe right. Your teacher will probably indicate when to inhale and exhale, but she won't let on that you're supposed to sound precisely like an overactive hot-water radiator. Practice this in your own home.

One must grunt, howl, and moan frequently in class, or others will think you are *not serious*.

Smoking cigarettes between pushups is frowned upon.

Snickering when a classmate trips and falls on her nose is absolutely verboten.

But you may wear a headband. This is the only time in life when you ever should.

HOW OFTEN?

Work out at least twice a week or you may just as well fester in that hammock. Three times a week is better. Your muscles get all zealous and enthusiastic when you start using them, they start humming little tunes and building new capillaries to carry the extra workload. But if you ignore them for 72 hours, muscles get discouraged and begin to atrophy. The capillaries dry up just like an old riverbed. It doesn't happen all at once; the average atrophy rate is 1 percent per day.

Do not get crazy and work out for hours every day or your muscles will just get tired and cranky. This syndrome is known as overtraining, and you'll start getting headaches, insomnia, and won't be able to eat or fuck.

HOW LONG?

If you're in a state of utter flaccidity and have no muscle tone to speak of, it will take you from eight to twelve months to develop into an Amazon. The older you are, the longer it takes. Be patient. Think of how long it took to build Rome. And you only need to do it for about five hours a week.

CELLULITE

Cellulite is no reason to put your head in the oven. More girls have cellulite than don't, and every one of them is convinced that her cellulite is probably the most nauseating in the Western Hemisphere.

Someone, somewhere, probably *does* have the worst cellulite in the Western Hemisphere, but chances are it isn't you.

Cellulite is a fancy word for dimpled fat, and French people have been making millions of dollars manufacturing products which prey on our insecurity about it. Exercise will reshape you and severely alleviate the flab effect, but only serious weight loss will completely cure cellulite, and looking like an Auschwitz victim is not necessarily appealing.

Your normal man doesn't mind cellulite nearly as much as you think, he's too busy worrying about his own lack of pectorals. So do your best to be casual and debonair about the whole cellulite business, or you'll find yourself backing out of rooms when naked and afraid to fuck in the shower. (Although I *would* stay away from overhead lighting, which just makes every single pucker stand out in sharp relief.)

SEX AND EXERCISE

It will come as no surprise to any of you that sex is the best exercise there is. One sweats, one pants, one utilizes the *entire* cardiovascular system. One's thighs become limber, one's pelvic girdle becomes obdurate.

But you can't just lie there. Make sure you get on top frequently, and do it in difficult, precarious positions that utilize the calf and thigh muscles—such as on top of the kitchen sink or while pretending to scrub the kitchen floor. Doing it in a chair is good, and hanging from a shower rod can be great for the triceps. Consult your physician first.

Having sex twice a day should be enough to keep you in shape—unless your lover suffers from premature ejaculation, in which case you'll have to do it four times.

CHEEKBONES AND ORAL SEX

Oral sex tunes up your masseter (jaw) muscles like nobody's business. Do it enough and you'll have positively Tartar cheekbones. If you can't find a man, you can always use an all-day sucker.

But most men will be pleased to oblige. You have to be careful though. Don't try it with your best friend's boyfriend, for example, or you may get a broken jaw instead.

SPORTS

Some sports will get you in shape, others won't.

If you play football, best to be a wide receiver or tight end, since they see so much action. If you play baseball, playing shortstop is infinitely preferable to pitching (ever noticed Fernando Valenzuela? A tub). Ice hockey is excellent but bad for the teeth. Any sort of martial art is wonderful, good for body and soul alike, and you won't have to carry mace in your handbag anymore, since once you get good at it you can break legs other than your own at a moment's notice.

BACKSLIDING

There will come a time during your newfound body consciousness when the thought of going back to your old slothful ways will seem laughable. "Who, me?" you'll say disdainfully. "*Me* go back to that lousy old hammock? Fat chance! I'm a new woman! I've seen the light! Have I shown you my triceps lately? I have? Would you like to see them again?"

And yet, letting things slide happens to the best of us. Anything can trigger this tragedy. An overdemanding job. A rotten love affair. A lingering virus. A new puppy.

Don't bother feeling guilty. The most industrious of girls, girls absolutely oozing with vim and vigor, will suddenly take to their beds until further notice.

Give yourself a bit of slack. Put exercising out of your mind for a week, two weeks, a month. Eventually your body will start clamoring for attention and you'll begin to pull yourself together. If all else fails, you can envision yourself on the beach next summer, which will get you up and moving in no time flat.

THE IMPORTANCE OF BEING RETICENT

Once you're physically fit, shut up about it. No one but your mother is interested in the state of your tendons. The girl who regales all and sundry on her methods of situps is a girl surrounded by people stifling yawns.

And be especially reticent in public places. When you decide to buy sneakers, do not ask the salesman in a loud voice what kind of turf this one or that one is good for. Let your teeming interest in turf remain in the closet.

And, now that we're on the subject, choose sneakers for aesthetic values only, since tender souls such as myself may have to look at your feet occasionally, and the colors of some of those awful running shoes make us cringe in pain and want to die.

And never, even on request, perform pushups at a party.

14

Outfits

"Several of the outfits, Ignatius noticed, were new enough and expensive enough to be properly considered offenses against taste and decency."
—A CONFEDERACY OF DUNCES
Every bit of clothing ought to make you pretty.
—IAN DURY

When it comes to selecting clothes, your unconscious has the best taste in the world. It knows what you need better than you do. It can tell if that strange greeny-yellow will make you look like an unripe banana or a woman of divine and tragic mystery. It knows that, with a waist like yours, you should never be caught dead in a dirndl.

The unconscious is a wonderful thing. Not only does it know about horizontal stripes making you look fatter, it also knows the secrets of the universe. It knows why the grass is green and dogs like to eat it. It knows why you crave Oreo cookies, why socks get lost in dryers, why the stars exist.

Of course it won't tell you, just like that. A very close-mouthed type, your unconscious. It holds onto secrets like a vise. Prying doesn't help. You can't sidle up to your unconscious and say, "So what's new, hon? Why do you think I bought that hideous shawl that makes me look like my own grandmother?" You can't even ask solicitously if it's feeling all right or would it like a nice glass of Stolichnaya. Your unconscious feels, and rightly so, that there are some things it must keep from you for your own good.

But in the clothes-choosing department, your unconscious goes too far. It does not seem fair that, unbeknown to you, every single item you put on your body literally shouts out your unconscious dreams and desires to the entire world. Everyone who sees you can read you like a book, yet you yourself have no idea what you're saying.

To combat this, look in mirrors every chance you get. Cultivate your mirror, think of it as your best friend. A little healthy narcissism is good for body and soul. Although staring fervently into the mirror for hours on end, forgetting hunger and the changing of the seasons, may be going too far. Just check yourself out whenever you're at home and have nothing more pressing to do.

(But never in public. Beau Brummell, that legendary Regency buck, used to spend hours in front of his bedroom mirror, perfecting the lines of his cravat, but when he emerged in public, he never gave a mirror even a sidelong glance. One simply didn't.)

As you stare into the mirror, take careful note of what you see. You will eventually discern that you are indeed projecting an image.

Here are some thumbnail sketches of certain images and what they are projecting to the populace at large. Perhaps you'll recognize yourself.

THE LITTLE GIRL

Pink is her wardrobe's middle name. Too much pink, in fact, is not enough. She is inordinately fond of pinafores and puffy sleeves, and has several pairs of anklets, many of them embroidered with teensy, darling little cornflowers. She may even call her dresses frocks, and not many of these frocks have waistlines, let alone a hint of cleavage. But almost all of them have frills dripping from at least one part of the garment, often the hemline or bodice. The

Little Girl is partial to sweet little prints and secretly wants to wear pigtails.

What the Little Girl is projecting is that she's still in the sandbox and therefore not responsible for anything. She spends most of her time looking for someone to take care of her, and although she can usually change a fuse faster than any truck driver, she's quick to disguise that knowledge.

The Little Girl is afraid of threatening *anyone* (probably had a bad relationship with her mother) and only feels comfortable when hiding her strength and sexuality.

The Little Girl doesn't get laid a whole lot. Men take a look at her and think, "Before I get her into bed, I'll probably have to paint her bathroom." And unless the man is truly smitten, he's going to find it daunting to wade through all those frills and furbelows to find out if she has the kind of body he likes. He may suspect she's hiding something.

But there is one kind of man drawn to the Little Girl like a lemming to the sea. No, not the big, strong construction worker looking for a little woman to protect. Her ardent admirer is the Little Boy. He'll realize that at last he's found his dream girl. They'll go to the zoo and cry over the baby polar bear. They'll write the New Wave version of *Peter Pan*. They'll play hopscotch. As a couple, no one will be able to stand them.

THE SEDUCTRESS

The Seductress likes to think she has a way with men, and she does. She knows that they like to see plenty of legs, plenty of tit, and jeans stretched tightly across a firm ass. Not only does she know this, she acts on it. One can find this woman in discount shops all over America, handling gold lamé and Spandex with a cool, appraising finger.

Often the Seductress is a waitress or barmaid, or else she's been seriously brainwashed. Waitresses and barmaids dress like this since even now it's usually men who leave tips. Seriously brainwashed women still look on men as their meal ticket.

Although the Seductress is often competitive with and downright surly to other women, it pays to cultivate her. Not only does she have vast stores of information about the proclivities and foibles of men, she also has a canny cynicism that is downright refreshing.

Men who are attracted to the Seductress are either simple, hard-working laborers or gangsters. Both like a flashy broad hanging off their arm—it gives them a sense of security, like a nice diamond pinky ring. But the Seductress has to be careful—not only will a man think her interchangeable with other Seductresses, he may also think her cheap—willing to perform fellatio after the first martini, never mind dinner. And football players will chase her down the street to propose assorted depravities.

THE DOMINATRIX

The Dominatrix wears black. Leather if possible. Nothing else will do.

No cuteness for her. She likes the clean, uncluttered look, a look rife with menace and danger and the possibility that she has a whip concealed about her person.

I myself stumbled upon this look by accident. This guy gave me a leather motorcycle jumpsuit that didn't fit him anymore. It was a work of primitive art, tough and black, with zippers everywhere.

Every time I wore this ominous creation, men flocked. Nice men too, not just weirdo sicko perverts. Sweet lawyers, innocent Country-and-Western singers, depressed dentists. That black leather and zippers drove them nuts.

I have no idea what this means. Most likely it has something to do with anger, the number one bugaboo of the '80s. Men especially have acres, miles, eons of anger—against news vendors who short-change them, against other guys who cut them off on highways, against everyone who wants their jobs, against uppity women demanding parity in work and love. But especially against themselves. They are rotten male chauvinist pigs and they know it. So they take one look at a girl in mean black leather and something inside them responds, they don't know what.

Be careful about this stuff. Sometimes men don't know whether you're kidding or not, and will really expect you to beat them up.

THE PREPPIE

As everyone knows, preppies are the scum of the earth. All except for my dearest friend Mary, the sweetest blonde on earth, who just happened to go to Vassar and never quite got over it.

The problem with Preppies is that they are obsessed with cotton. Now, all of us are fond of the stuff, but when the right alligator on the right pocket is of such staggering significance, we're talking fascism.

Preppie girls attract only Preppie boys and crazy artists craving humiliation. A Preppie's image states to all concerned that sex is the furthest thing from her mind, something well below the interest level of her golf handicap. No man figures that a Preppie actually *likes* sex, but he hopes that if he's a very good boy indeed, she just may deign to give him a hand job.

DESIGNER LABEL GIRL

The DLG is an insecure girl in the grip of a massive identity crisis. Her scarves, shoes, handbags, even sunglasses, have initials on them other than her own, a situation that unnerves even the strongest. A DLG doesn't care what she looks like as long as she looks expensive. She will wear red with orange and not notice.

Consciously the DLG is trying to project that she's got cash and chic and plenty of both, but her unconscious is singing a completely different tune.

"I have no idea who I am," the DLG is projecting, "so could you please remind me?"

The men she attracts will tell her all right. With that first glance at the YSL on her lapel, the sadistic sort of man can tell he's got a live one. "No sense of herself," he'll muse sinisterly. "I think I'll treat her like a dog. I think I'll make her wash my windows while I'm off cavorting with an airline stewardess."

Listen here, DLG: If you want to be treated fairly, never wear anyone's initials but your own. (No, not even a discreet "G" on the buckle of your shoe. No, not even an almost indiscernible "Dior" woven into the fabric of your nightgown.)

THE HIPPIE

Once upon a time, everyone who was anyone was a hippie, although they didn't call themselves that. As Arlo Guthrie said, "There was about six months there in 1966 when you could tell who had a roach in his pocket just by what he was wearing."

Alas, we are now well into the '80s, and what used to mean that one was ready to go anywhere, do anything, take any drug and sleep with all and sundry now means that you bake your own bread and breastfeed your baby.

The Hippie's wardrobe is deeply homespun. Shawls and denim and blouses from India with mirrors all over them are her mainstays, but occasionally she'll branch out into an Afghani coat.

A Hippie attracts businessmen, graduate students, and other hippies. A businessman still thinks that she will give him all the free love he wants, and will laugh at her efforts to feed him granola.

THE CORPORATE DRESSER

If you happen to be one of those women who believe in pinstriped, A-line-skirted suits with vests, you are reading the wrong book. Put it down immediately and go back to your annual report.

Once you realize what your image is, get rid of it. Clothes are the mirror of the soul, and your soul, as you know, is multifaceted, multileveled, and too complex for words. You can't stick to one look when one second you feel like Emily Dickinson and the next like Bette Midler.

Instead of dressing for the image, dress for the *moment*. This is not a concept to be taken lightly. The right combination of clothes can make or break your minute, day, life. One must, under every circumstance, be dressed appropriately. (Okay, you can run out to the corner for cigarettes in *anything*. Except if you happen to be crazy about someone who lives down the block, which happened to me once. What a nightmare, twenty minutes choosing the perfect T-shirt. Thank God he moved uptown.)

Dressing appropriately doesn't mean gray slacks to the supermarket and silk dresses for lunch with men. Dressing appropriately means that your outfit makes you feel like singing a little song and dancing a peppy jig.

Penny, my crazy rock-star friend, likes to reminisce about the old days when she would fly to Boston in a silver batwinged minidress, a black leather silver-studded aviator's helmet, purple vinyl trench coat, and fishnet stockings.

"Sounds pretty pretentious to me," I told her.

"So what?" she said. "I felt like the fucking Queen of the May. I felt like a million bucks. Isn't that the point?"

That is, in fact, the point. So get yourself some wonderful clothes.

HOW TO SHOP

1. *Lie down.*

When embarking on anything major, it's always a good idea to be prone. Daydream a little. Fantasize. Play around. Put on a record. This activity will enable your unconscious to unbutton its lip a little, and eventually it will come to you that, although you seem to spend all your time wearing tweedy suits because of your job at the university, what you really want is a great big red velour jump suit with a nipped-in waist.

2. *Keep this image firmly in mind.*

Don't let go of what you want and how you want to look for a second. This is essential when entering a shop, because many an undecided girl has fallen prey to those deeply cunning salesgirls who populate finer boutiques all over the country.

You know the ones I mean. They've all got long, straight, artfully cut blond hair and they're always wearing a certain perfect something and have absolutely no hips. They look as if they just flew in from France or Milan on the Concorde and are only helping out in the shop for a lark so they'll have something to giggle about over a trendy little lunch with their friends Monique and Daniela. ("My God, Daniela, you wouldn't *believe* the mutant who came in today! She must have had a *twenty-six*-inch waist!")

This creature is to be avoided like an insurance salesman. Which won't be easy, since the minute you walk into the shop she'll pretend you're her long-lost sister. She'll spout endearing words at you in a French accent, and if you're not careful you'll start saying *Très bien* to her. She may even hug you as she steers you to a stunningly weird and catastrophically expensive rack of dresses just arrived from Tokyo.

"This is the dress of the season," she'll tell you, "so *chic*, so *je ne sais quoi*. And it will set your waist off to perfection."

Say what? What waist? You look behind you, thinking that she must be talking to someone else. But no, now she's herding you inexorably toward the dressing room, her hand encircling your wrist like a steel handcuff.

3. *Remember Lester Bangs.*

Lester was a lunatic and brilliant writer who once said, "Style is originality; fashion is fascism. The two are eternally and unalterably opposed." Remember these blindingly trenchant words as you're being dragged to the dressing room with a state-of-the-art dress from Tokyo, and revolt.

Simply grab the salesgirl's thumb and pull it backward until she lets go, at which point you can say, very nicely, "No, thank you, *chérie*, the dress is perfectly heavenly and obviously the *dernier cri* in fashion, but I couldn't care a button. What I'm really interested in is that snappy red jump suit over there on the sale rack."

She'll act as if a spider had just fallen down her slender back, but the hell with her. You know who you are, she doesn't.

Another thing you've got to watch about salesgirls, even those nice, relaxed ones who don't work on commission, is that they're always trying to get you to belt things.

There you'll be in front of the mirror, trying to see what a dress would look like without a huge alarm-tag wadded at the hem, and the salesgirl will be at your side insisting that it looks great but would look *so* much better belted. Then she'll run off and return with some horrible eyesore of a belt and make you put it on, which will only confuse and irritate you to the point that you inadvertently buy the dress.

When you get it home, you'll find that without the alarm-tag the belt just makes it look all bunchy, and without the belt it hangs abysmally. You'll decide that maybe the belt isn't really so bad after all and hang the dress in your closet, where it will fester for two years and eventually be given to your cousin, who won't wear it either.

4. *Only buy something you're seriously in love with.*

The garment in question should jump off the hanger, throw its arms around your neck and shout, "I'm for you." Wait for this. Don't get impatient and settle for mere infatuation, because the moment you take the approximation home, those pearl buttons you thought would probably be okay will reveal themselves as the atrocities they really are.

The closets of most women are paved with good intentions. Often you feel as if you ought to have a blouse with pearl buttons because Agnes in accounting looks terrific in hers, but refrain. Either you're a pearl-button girl or you're not.

5. *Don't let a prettily phrased price turn your head.*

Okay, so this Armani blazer has been marked down from $700 to $29.95. So what? Twenty-nine ninety-five is still enough for a decent lunch, which will fare you a lot better than an Armani blazer with a sleeve length that makes you look like a gorilla.

6. *Shop a lot.*

A good three or four hours of shopping will alleviate all but the heaviest anxiety attack, especially if you don't need to buy anything.

Also, shopping a lot can prevent painful mistakes. Sometimes your taste will play tricks on you. You'll fall crazily in love with oh, say, a blue jacket and think it's the very thing for you to wear every day for the rest of your life. Then, if you start shopping around, you may see that blue jacket everywhere—displayed in store windows, festooned over glass counters, adorning every third girl on the street. You'll wonder what you ever saw in the damned thing. No one knows what causes this phenomenon, but it probably has something to do with food additives.

7. *Keep away from polyester.*

There's something sinister about polyester. Oh, I know, easy-care, no ironing, all that. But there is strong evidence that it makes the brain cells fuse, and that years of wearing the stuff amounts to the same thing as having a prefrontal lobotomy. Possibly this isn't true, but don't risk it. Even more important, polyester infuses its wearer with a vague feeling of inferiority. This is because almost all polyester is pretending to be something else, usually silk. People, glancing from afar, may even think it *is* silk. But you, dear wearer, will know the sordid truth, and this knowledge will make you despondent.

8. *Buy classy items.*

You'll feel much better wearing a well-stitched, carefully crafted garment than some piece of sleaze that just looks good on the outside. Even if only you know that it's real Harris tweed, you will still exude that special air which will give the merest passerby the feeling that you're someone special, possibly that actress she saw this morning on the "Today" show.

If you're rich, it's easy. If not, haunt thrift stores. Church rummage sales in rural areas are veritable gold mines. But do try to stay away from ornate period pieces that make you look like a runaway from a wax museum.

9. *You need only three pairs of shoes.*

Black boots, white sneakers, and red heels—all else is gravy.

The boots should have the soft sheen of good leather, and, current fashions notwithstanding, the heels should not be so flat that your ankles look dumpy. But you should be able to run in them if you have to.

Do not even think about making do with vinyl; these are your actual feet we're talking about. Feet need to feel pampered and loved or they'll turn on you just when you need them the most.

White sneakers do not have to be some fancy hundred-dollar brand, although those in the bargain basement of five-and-dimes have an alarming tendency to mangle your little toe.

Okay, you don't have to have red heels, but they work for me. Every time. The angels want to wear them, but I won't let them. When you're wearing red heels, you dance like Carmen Miranda and sing like Billie Holiday. They have soul, red shoes. They make you jaunty and jolly.

But be careful; other girls will be overcome with jealousy and try to rip them off your feet. Mysterious strangers with melting blue eyes will try to follow you home. Cowboys will automatically assume you can two-step. Certain schoolteachers will try to have you arrested.

And never, ever, wear trendy, complicated shoes. Eschew shoes riddled with silver studs, plastic bows, silver ribbons, or anything even remotely adorable. They look self-conscious, and when they're exceedingly trendy, they'll be out of fashion as soon as you wear them to the corner.

Who can ever forget the fall of '81, when nine out of ten girls spent an entire week's paycheck on a pair of up-to-the-second metallic ankle boots? And who can forget the winter of '81–'82, when all those girls shamefacedly hid these monstrosities way in the back of their closets? And who can forget the spring of '82, when every second-hand shop had a special on metallic ankle boots, two pairs 25¢?

Comfort is crucial. If you're going to spend a week's paycheck, you want to wear your shoes for a bit. When you try them on in a shop, parade around in them until the salesperson starts yawning and giving you fishy glances. When you're absolutely sure they don't hurt anywhere and have studied them carefully to confirm the absence of cunning little bows, walk around in them for another half hour. Never think that you'll break them in and they'll be just fine. I personally just gave the Salvation Army six pair of the cutest shoes ever. I pity the poor women who purchase them. By the bye, patent leather is the worst. It never stretches a micrometer, and it gives Catholic schoolboys some very strange notions.

Shoes with holes at the toe are only okay if you have a beautifully formed and impeccably varnished big toe.

High-heeled, thin-strapped sandals have been known to drive some men to frenzies, but they're often men who want to tie you up, so be careful.

Silicone sprays don't let leather breathe, turning it virtually into vinyl.

It is exceedingly passé to worry about having big feet. Nobody who's anybody wants dainty feet anymore. Let them be as big as they want. Marta, a femme fatale if ever there was one, decided her feet weren't comfortable enough, so she started buying size nines, what the hell. Her feet are eternally grateful.

DRESSING FOR MEN

Once, when I was a lucky young journalist, I got to interview Walter Matthau, a real sweetheart. Something about me struck a paternalistic chord, and he kept stopping the interview to call his brothers and cousins to see if they knew a good fellow for me.

Then, at one point, he looked me over carefully and shook his head sadly. I thought I looked pretty great in my regulation baseball uniform top and multifrilled plaid skirt, but Walter wasn't having it.

"You look like some kind of Gilda-Radner-Saturday-Night-Live beatnik," he said mournfully, in that special tone he has. "You'll never get laid, looking like that. What you need is a simple black dress, sort of 'forties style, and get your goddamned hair up and out of the way."

"The hell with him," I thought, all my feminist zeal rearing its imperious head.

But secretly, without telling anyone, I did what he said and immediately noticed a strong upsurge in male attention.

If you want sex, you have to present yourself in a sexually appetizing manner. This does *not* mean dressing for men, it simply means dressing with your sexuality in mind.

Which works better anyway. Nobody ever knows what a man is going to find sexy. They say for Elvis Presley it was white cotton panties. For the lawyer who lives upstairs from me, it's anklets with high heels. It's true that men are pretty cut-and-dried in their lingerie tastes, a subject we'll be getting to in a moment, but otherwise they're obstreperous devils.

Although most of them like a bit of body curve showing, and 97 percent of them like high heels, and all of them like black. Always remember to have a little black something in your closet, cleaned and pressed and happy, so that when out of nowhere some perfectly fascinating specimen of manhood wants to come over and profess undying love, you've got something to wear.

One more thing. Shoulder pads, in my opinion, are the greatest thing humankind ever devised. They make you look skinny. They make you look mysterious. They make you look like you're just about to say, "You know how to whistle, don't you? Just put your lips together and blow."

But otherwise, don't take anybody's word for anything. Just wear whatever you think is achingly sexy. You're bound to find a fellow who will agree wholeheartedly.

LETTING GO

There comes a time in every girl's life when it is psychologically imperative to dispense with all thoughts of clothes and image. One never knows when the thought of washing one's hair, plucking one's eyebrows, and finding the perfect socks will plunge one into deep, irretrievable melancholy.

Sometimes too much attention to self makes one feel victimized. When this feeling comes on, it is intransigent. You could be in the midst of a fascinating affair with a man who inspires you to don all sorts of frilly off-the-shoulder dresses because something about him, you don't know what, makes you feel all sweet and feminine, and then suddenly a cold dread will wash over you at the sight of a silk camisole.

Ignore this feeling at your peril. Get your body immediately into some nice, soft, comfortable jeans and tattered sweatshirt. Eschew makeup, don't wash your hair.

This will feel great, a lot like the way our foremothers felt when taking off their corsets of an evening. If your man doesn't like it, fuck him. Then he'll either like it fine or he's some kind of lame-brain who doesn't expect you to be the multifaceted enigma that you are. If he doesn't like it, he doesn't have to look at you. He can read a book.

Eventually you will want to pretty yourself up again, but don't rush it, you've got years to spare.

15

Lingerie Do's and Don'ts

Always remember that lingerie is not clothes. Clothes have a utilitarian purpose. They keep you warm and dry, they do their best to camouflage body flaws. They provide pockets in which you can keep money, an answering-machine beeper, mace, your diaphragm. (Have I ever mentioned the time that Laura, a creative-theology student, went to a nightclub with her diaphragm rolled into the sleeve of her T-shirt? A symbolic gesture if there ever was one.)

But lingerie has no purpose whatsoever except for sex. Well, yes, a bra keeps your breasts lined up with the darts of your blouse, and the cotton crotch of your panties prevents you from getting vaginal infections, but we're not talking underwear here. We're talking slips, petticoats, camisoles, teddies, tap pants, garters, garter belts, stockings, negligees, pushup bras, bloomers, corsets, and G-strings.

Depending on your body type, you should always have on hand several samples of the above.

When buying lingerie, think filthy thoughts, and think about men. And don't think you're some kind of nonfeminist disgusting reactionary sniveling turncoat for doing this, because you're not. Turning a man on as much as possible is beneficial to both concerned.

Even in the lingerie department, men are a bit unpredictable. Some like you to look all white and dewy and virginal (usually Catholics). Others (usually Catholics) like you to look as if you just stepped out of a sleazy New Orleans bordello. One man told me once that he likes striped underwear because the stripes suggest imprisonment. (I suddenly remembered an urgent appointment.)

So buy whatever makes you feel like the hottest number in town. Wearing the right panties can be as sexually crucial as having terrific legs. These panties will inevitably make you feel like Evelyn Nesbit on a good day. If they don't, throw them out.

—Be aware that *only extremely perverted and downright sicko men like pantyhose.* Men who like pantyhose have been known to strangle innocent old ladies for no reason. And not only that, but they don't have the slightest idea how to fuck. Well, they have a vague idea, and it entails getting on top of you for a moment or two and concentrating fervently on baseball statistics. Then they roll off and fall asleep with their mouths open.

—*Stockings and garter belts are essential.* They make you feel all femme-fatalish, like a woman who knows what's what but isn't telling, like a woman who's had a hit song written for her. Plus they're practical—pantyhose are notorious breeding grounds for the dread trichomoniasis bacteria.

Equip yourself with two black and one novelty garter belt. By novelty I mean something pink and tenuous, or possibly sleek flesh-toned satin. You will not be needing a garter belt festooned with funny jokes or the days of the week.

—*Stockings should not be orange.* In fact, nothing you wear should ever be orange, a singularly hideous color. (Rita vehemently disputes this, and is always throwing long orange scarves around her neck and looking fine. Maybe you have to be a six-foot-one redhead to get away with it.)

Black, that's the ticket, especially in the stocking department. Black won't let you down.

Think about Anna Magnani in *The Rose Tattoo*. She looked pretty dumpy, old Anna, until she appeared in a black lace slip, which immediately transformed her into a woman of unspeakable and intriguing desires.

Fishnet stockings are nice if you're in a cheap and tawdry mood.

Patterned stockings are often a hit, although one shouldn't go mental and wear a pair with green and purple swirls all over them. And all stockings should be long enough, otherwise you have to pull your garter belt down so far that you'll cut off all circulation in your ass, which, when not numb, is a powerful erogenous zone.

Stockings should also be roomy at the top or they'll make your thighs bulge out. Men don't mind this thigh bulge, but still. Actually, sometimes a man likes this thigh bulge too much and starts slavering and whining like a Doberman confronting a burglar. If this happens, a pitcher of ice water will quell his gibbering.

Seamed stockings aren't subtle, but they certainly do the job. You shouldn't wear them when out with someone you're not prepared to sleep with, since their presence is tantamount to saying, "Hi there, big fellow, please rip my clothes off at your earliest opportunity." If you really want your escort paralytic with lust, stop frequently to adjust the seams. But never wear them with flat shoes, it doesn't work.

If you can find stockings with a bit of discreet embroidery on the ankle, snap them up. They've been known to stop traffic.

—*Panties go on top of garter belts.* Never the other way around, or the whole works have to come off before you have sex.

—*A bit of camouflage is permissible.* If you have bad thighs or a droopy ass, try long Victorian bloomers or tap pants, which look good on anyone who has a waist. If you have small breasts, lacy camisoles are perfect. But don't wear a camisole if you're generously endowed, you'll just look bovine. If you don't have a waist, you may want to dabble in corsets.

Do not get carried away with camouflage. A wonderfully free, open and fulfilling sexual relationship cannot blossom and flower if you refuse to be seen naked.

—*Never spend $60 for antique silk underwear.* Old silk rips in a second. Normal wear and tear with your average lust-crazed fellow is three minutes, tops. He may adore tearing the stuff off you, but you'll forget to notice.

"Oh, darling, it's so wonderful," he'll be saying.

"Sixty dollars down the fucking drain," you'll be muttering.

This is what we call cross-purposes.

—*The best thing to do.* When someone riveting asks you out, tell him that you'd like to meet early, like in the afternoon, for a drink. Make sure the bar you choose is near a great lingerie store.

Have a few margaritas and drag him off shopping.

Now a man alone in a lingerie shop is a sorry creature to behold— he gets red and stammers and is absolutely certain that the smiling saleswoman is convinced he actually wants that purple lace garter belt for himself. Usually he trips and lands face down in the panty display and has to be led, firmly and gently, out the door.

But a man in a lingerie shop with a woman is a smug fellow indeed. He gives all and sundry a jaunty smile, a smile which, if it spoke, would inform the world that he is a hell of a guy, a devil with the ladies, the sort of fellow whom women drag into lingerie shops every chance they get.

He'll be in a sunny mood as you pick up a lace corset and ask him what he thinks. He'll start getting a bit excited when you tell him to wait a second while you try on a minuscule French pushup bra. By the time you start wondering about the feasibility of a G-string, his mind will be calculating furiously, trying to figure out how to get out of going to the movies and getting you immediately to a suite at the Plaza, where he can study your purchases at leisure, at length.

Which reminds me of the time I got Jake to take me to Frederick's of Hollywood, home of the crotchless panty and nippleless bra.

Astute readers will remember that Jake is that wonderful fellow whom I fled from for no reason at all, except that he loved me when I was convinced I was a toad.

Frederick's of Hollywood wasn't what I expected. It is presided over by kindly, middle-aged women who discuss the merits of peekaboo bras the way many women discuss meatloaf recipes.

"Well, hon," one said to me, "I would get this fuchsia pushup bra here, accentuating your cleavage the way it does, and it complements that garter belt beautifully. A very appetizing combination."

Jake was very quiet as we drove back to his house.

"I thought you said we were going to stop somewhere to eat," I said, my purchases nestled in my lap.

"Well, we're not," he growled. "It's time to go home."

"But I'm hungry."

"No you're not."

"I'm not?"

"You know damned well you're not, so cut it out. We're not stopping anywhere. We're going straight home and when we get there you're not going to get on the phone or turn on the TV or decide to make a grilled cheese sandwich. We're going straight to my room and you're going to put all that stuff on and I'm going to take it off, piece by piece. And we're not going to leave the bedroom until I'm good and ready. Okay?"

See? It really works.

16

How to Be Blindingly Beautiful

Every woman in the world, even one with utterly no chin, has within her the capacity to be blindingly beautiful, to look younger than she ever dreamed in her wildest dreams.

But there is one simple rule you must follow:

Never lead a sensible life.

The moment you decide that you're a grownup now, and therefore must put away foolish things like staying out all night or cruising down strange highways is the moment you will lose that ineffable glow of youth.

If you don't believe me, look around. Study those people who would rather go to shopping malls than dance halls, who think the height of depravity is bidding two no trump with only fifteen points. Every single one of these people has a stringy neck.

Show me a woman who is prouder of her clean kitchen than of her collection of lingerie and I'll show you a woman with enlarged pores.

I know a forty-three-year-old newspaper editor who looked twenty-eight and never had split ends until she moved to the suburbs of Washington and immersed herself in cocktail parties and car pools. Within days, her hair lost its shine and crow's-feet appeared around her eyes.

"It was uncanny," she told me. "Suddenly I was this awful old frump. I told my husband we had to move back into the city, and fast. He was annoyed at first, but when I got cute again he perked up."

It's true for men, too. I know a man, a forty-five-year-old innkeeper, who brought up three children and drank a case of beer a day while doing so. This man is so handsome that Bruce Springsteen would shrink from being in the same room with him. It wasn't always so. This innkeeper showed me a snapshot once.

"Who's that fat oaf with the ridiculous vandyke beard?" I asked.

"Why, that's me," he said, "when I was practicing corporate law. I hated practicing corporate law, but I thought it was the adult thing to do. But eventually I couldn't stand it and thought what the hell, I'll move to Vermont. Much more fun."

If you want to keep your looks, cultivate the following characteristics:

—*Think about sex constantly*. Always wish you were having some. If fifteen minutes goes by and you haven't had some outlandish sexual fantasy, start worrying.

—*Do not stop listening to rock-and-roll*. Rock-and-roll withdrawal is more destructive to one's looks than severe overexposure to sun. And not just the Beatles, either. You have to listen to groups who still exist. Good Country-and-Western music (not that soppy string-riddled stuff) is equally rejuvenating.

—*Never be absolutely positive that your entire life won't suddenly do a backflip*. If your existence is plotted out for years in front of you—day by day, week by week, coffee spoon by coffee spoon—you will inevitably grow jowls.

—*Never decline excitement*. The girl who refuses to climb a tall fence to go skinny-dipping in the moonlight is the girl who will soon be needing bifocals.

—*Make sure you love somebody*. It doesn't have to be romantic love, although that is optimum. Even loving a cousin or a best friend will keep the skin soft and pleasant. Lack of love gives you creases at the corners of your mouth and a furrowed forehead.

—*Avoid excessive avarice and greed*. If you exist only to hang golden nuggets around your neck and string Bentleys down your driveway, you may as well check into an old age home.

"Enough," I hear you say, "of the cosmology. Bring on the cosmetology! What about moisturizers? What about hair care?"

HAIR CARE

Hair, being a secondary sex characteristic and therefore of crucial importance, must be treated with reverential respect. Pamper it, coddle it, pay close attention to its whims, give it its space.

Keep it clean. Never think to yourself, "I have dry hair, so I won't wash it for a week and maybe some oil will ooze into it." And don't get more convoluted and think, "I have oily hair, so maybe if I don't wash it for a week the oil glands won't be stimulated and will settle down."

Wash your hair every day with mild shampoo. Dilute the shampoo, since most of them on the market are too surly and abrasive. Cheap shampoos usually have the least harmful additives. Use a mild-mannered conditioner.

"And comb your hair, don't brush it," says Rita. "If your hair is tangled, do not have a temper tantrum and rip it apart or you will begin to resemble a Zulu warrior."

(I have Rita and Cleo here to throw beauty tips my way. Although I don't know how much help they'll be, since they persist in talking about men. No, now they're talking about horses, even worse. Wait, now we're back to men. On horses. I will slap their hands.)

"Blondes should always rinse their hair in camomile," says Cleo, snapping out of it for the nonce.

"Everyone should try being a blonde once in her life," says Rita, who is a redhead. "They have more fun since you can usually find them in the dark."

Ahem. Well, if you want to be a blonde, don't have your entire head bleached or the dark roots will begin to show in approximately seven minutes and you'll have to visit your hair colorist after every meal.

Have your hair subtly highlighted instead. It will last for months. No great big clumps of yellow—and eschew that suburban-lady effect of platinum streaks against very dark hair.

"Never dye your hair purple or something," says Cleo. "If you crave sudden weird color, use one of those washable sprays instead. But purple is passé anyway."

Don't worry about things being passé. If a certain hair effect makes you feel like the juiciest thing to come along since Helen of Troy, let no fashion clone deflect you.

Especially do not listen to fashion magazines. I happen to know for a fact that they haven't a clue.

"What shall we tell everyone to do with their hair this month?" the beauty editor of every fashion magazine is always wailing at editorial meetings.

"Who the hell knows?" mutters the shoe editor, who figures it's not her department anyway.

"Let's get them to look like wild, untamed tigresses," pipes up a hot-to-trot assistant editor.

"No, we did that last month," says the beauty editor.

"Sleek, sculptured goddesses?" hazards the fiction editor.

"The month before last," says the beauty editor sadly. "Oh, what the hell, let's just tell them to cut it all off."

"Always have long hair so you can flip it at men," says Rita.

You needn't have long hair, but under no circumstances affect a middle-aged-lady hairdo. You know the one. It's an inch and a half all around, has no shape, and makes the prettiest girl look like a linebacker.

In fact, keep away from hairdos altogether. A hairdo, by definition, always makes you look like someone else. Or think you do. I shall never forget that period in the late '70s when half the female population was scurrying around in a Farrah Fawcett-do while the other half was making do with the Dorothy Hamill-do.

"Who's Dorothy Hamill?" asks Cleo.

The best way to make sure you don't have a hairdo is to study yourself carefully in the mirror and ascertain that you don't remind yourself of anyone.

Try cutting your hair yourself at least once, just in case you can do it. If you can, you will save years of anguish, humiliation, and money.

The easiest haircut to give yourself is a sort of layered, just-got-out-of-bed cut. Grab some handy nail scissors, take small clumps from the top of your head, cut them one to three inches long. As you work your way down, cut the clumps longer, leaving it pretty much alone at the bottom.

"You can't do that with straight hair," says Rita.

Well you can, but it's a bit precarious. This technique is best with thick, wavy hair.

But you probably won't be able to cut your hair yourself.

HOW TO FIND A HAIRDRESSER

—Do not go to that convenient little shop around the corner. It may be easy, but you won't really enjoy looking like Queen Elizabeth on a bad day.

—If you see someone with a stunning haircut, grab her by the wrist and demand fiercely to know the name, address, and home phone number of her hairdresser. If she refuses to tell you, burst into tears.

—If you live in a city where magazines are published, check the fine print next to a haircut you like to find the name of the hairdresser. Then call him at his salon and tell him you're the pretender to the throne of Yugoslavia. Hairdressers have to be outrageously snobbish or they get thrown out of the hairdressing union. The hairdressing union meets every morning and all the members report how they had an emergency call from Brooke Shields at 5 A.M. If the pretender-to-the-throne routine doesn't work, sniff loudly over the phone and intimate that you're a prominent cocaine dealer. You'll get an appointment.

—Keep away from a hairdresser you can bully. Any hairdresser who will let you bring in a magazine clipping and tell him you want it exactly like that is a hairdresser to be shunned.

—Avoid straight male hairdressers. Straight men always have an ideal woman in mind, and will cut every woman's hair accordingly. Often the straight male hairdresser's ideal is Cheryl Tiegs, and he will do his best to make you fit the mold. Nobody in her right mind wants to look like Cheryl Tiegs—all that rampant wholesomeness— in fact, one often wonders how Cheryl Tiegs can stand looking in the mirror every morning. "Oh, God, there I am again!" she must cry to herself.

"I like Cheryl Tiegs," Rita says, which proves that Texans are weird.

—Stick to women or gay men. They will identify with you. They will know what you mean when you say you want to look like a cross between a royal duchess and a fifty-dollar-a-night hooker.

—Observe the hairdresser closely. Make sure he's looking at you, not himself, in the mirror. That he studies the texture of your hair and notes the way it falls. He should not cut your hair when it's sopping wet. If he recommends a permanent or straightening, be exceedingly haughty.

How to Control Your Hairdresser

"Never cry," says Rita.

"Always cry," says Cleo.

"When he says, 'Who cut your hair last, Godzilla?' tell him sweetly that he did, two months ago," says Rita.

"Tell him if he doesn't make you beautiful you'll tell his mother where he was on Monday night," says Cleo.

And always, if you plan on going back, give him an enormous tip. Nothing stirs the creative juices like a little lucre.

SKIN CARE

Skin, like Greta Garbo, often craves a lot less attention than it gets. Especially if you are under twenty-five, when you should simply wash it and forget about it. If you have pimples, go to a dermatologist.

"But not one of those dermatologists who thinks it might be fun to start excavating your face," says Cleo. "I actually have a scar from one of those sadists."

After twenty-five, you have to decide if your skin is dry or oily. If it's dry, you have to wash it with creamy soap and use a moisturizer or you'll be wrinkled by the time you're thirty. Especially when venturing into the sun or wind.

"And if you don't know that by now, you're a Martian," says Rita.

If you have oily skin, you still have to put cream around your eyes and on your upper lip, but you should only use water-based foundation and no moisturizer except in abovementioned areas. Moisturizers just clog oily skin and make it sag. Mainly keep it clean. Use sterilized cotton with your astringent, use fresh towels, wash your makeup brushes. Otherwise you'll get blackheads, which, although striking, are not appealing.

Do not bother to have facials. Even if a facial is done properly it's not much good, but when it's done wrong it can stretch your skin and make it fall in folds off your face.

"And stay away from those fancy skin mavens," says Rita. "One doesn't wish to name names, but anyone who sells you a bottle of cleansing oil for twenty-seven dollars is only having her little joke, and the joke's on you. I used to go to one of them, and whenever I needed new supplies I had to give up drink and drugs for a month. A dermatologist charges about one-third the price for better products."

"To tighten pores, use a sperm mask," says Cleo. "Just before he's about to come, point the penis toward your cheek. Rub the ejaculate into your skin in smooth upward motions. Leave on for five minutes. Remove with cool water splashed lightly on the face. Your skin will be tight, well nourished, sexually satisfied."

"Ignore that deranged woman," says Rita. "Use tea bags on your eyes when you have a hangover, reduces puffiness."

"I prefer cucumber," says Cleo. "Also, if you don't have any sperm, you can use egg white to tighten pores. Store it in a closed container in your refrigerator. Smooth gently on the face. Repeat procedure as for sperm."

MAKEUP TIPS

Makeup, much like Greta Garbo, should never actually be seen, but should retain its mystery. Eye shadow should never be slathered on lids. Blusher should never be applied in hard, decisive lines under the mistaken impression that it makes one look like Lauren Hutton. Mascara should not transform the eyelashes into iron filings. And lipstick, when applied too thickly, is unseemly and inevitably ends up on your front teeth.

During the day, be reticent with makeup unless you're planning to spend your time stationary on a sofa. This is not a bad idea, but most modern girls find that they must run hither and yon— going to the post office, dropping off the laundry, taking over multinational corporations. The more makeup you wear, the more chance that by the end of the day your blusher will be smeared across your nose, your mascara will have formed two thick black crescents under your eyes, and your lips will be a kidney-shaped blur.

During the evening, however, use as much makeup as you want to. Sometimes even more than you want to. I did that once and—

"Oh, my God," Cleo is groaning, "we're in for one of her *stories*."

"Make it short, darlin'," Rita says. "Your readers are busy women."

I was just going to say that sometimes, when you're especially attracted to a man, you purposely tone yourself down. "No, you think to yourself, I won't wear that fabulous dress with the slit up the side, he'll think I'm trying too hard. And I'd better cool it with the eye liner."

Well, one night I had a bit part in a play and was forced to wear heavy stage makeup when meeting this adorable architect for dinner.

"Wasn't that the one you went off to Monte Carlo with?" Cleo asks.

I have never been to Monte Carlo in my life, she is only kidding. Suffice to say, however, that it sometimes behooves a girl to be bold and daring.

And yet, still subtle. Show strong confidence, but never use a heavy hand. Subtlety is the soul of seduction.

"Which means," says Cleo, "that there is nothing more hideous than heavy, thick, disgusting pancake makeup slathered on the face."

"And if you have light skin don't decide to give yourself an artificial suntan by applying foundation a dozen shades darker," says Rita.

"Everyone knows that," says Cleo.

"I wish they did," Rita says sadly.

Never paint flowers on your face, or put decals on your nails.

Use brown instead of black eye liner under the eyes and you will look less like a raccoon.

Smooth splotchy blusher with a tissue.

Line the lips before coloring them, then blot.

Never pluck eyebrows beyond the inner corner of the eye.

Use pale-blue eye shadow only if you wish to resemble a sorority girl.

Try your best to keep away from orange lipstick.

Experiment madly in the privacy of your home. Have beauty makeovers, even those silly ones they give you at department stores, since an impartial observer may come up with a few ideas you've never thought about, and may even be able to tell you that mauve eye shadow makes you look macabre and not ethereal like you thought.

Eventually, of course, you will begin to wrinkle, no matter how frivolous a life you lead. When a woman reaches the age where a man of the same age would be called "rugged," she should stop using all but the most rudimentary makeup. An older woman is just as attractive and sexy as an older man as long as she is proud of her wrinkles and doesn't seem to be cowering behind heavy camouflage. One must never apply eye liner over crow's-feet.

HAIR REMOVAL

Do not even think of shaving your eyebrows.

Cream hair removers are smelly and horrid and not worth the bother.

Waxing one's legs and underarms causes several seconds of intense pain, but then you don't have to do anything for approximately six weeks. Waxing of one's "bikini area" is so painful that it's not worth it unless you're exceptionally hirsute or exceptionally vain.

"And electrolysis of the bikini area should only be attempted under general anesthesia," says Cleo.

Electrolysis is always painful, and anyone who tries to tell you differently is nursing a secret grudge. Plus you have to keep going back, since they never get all those unsightly hairs the first, or even second, time around. But once it's done, it's done. I am supremely jealous of my friend Mary, who will never have to pluck another eyebrow as long as she lives.

KEEPING CLEAN

The only girls who are allowed not to shower every day are Europeans and girls in the final stages of depression.

You may of course bathe instead. If you do, do not spend fifteen dollars on fancy bath oil which only lasts for four and a half baths. Mix baby oil with your perfume.

Deodorant soaps should not be countenanced.

Flossing of the teeth may not be done where anyone can watch you.

Frequent toothbrushing is good for the gums and not considered bourgeois or reactionary. Soft bristles only.

"What about douching?" wonders Rita.

"Trust *you* to lower the tone," says Cleo.

Douching should never be performed more than twice a week unless your doctor tells you to. Keep away from herbal, fruity, floral, or other such twee douches. Vinegar and water will suffice and will help curb infections—two tablespoons per quart of warm water.

"You can tell you have a vaginal infection if you smell like ammonia, sourdough bread, or an old mackerel," says Cleo.

"Who's lowering the tone *now?*" Rita wants to know.

Steer clear of deodorant tampons, deodorant sanitary napkins, and other such muck.

"And do not spray cologne on sensitive labial tissues," says Rita, wincing.

Remember that normal vaginal odor is normal, and Mother Nature, in her infinite wisdom, gave it to us for a reason. Back in primeval times, men liked it. Some filthy perverts still do.

BEAUTY FEEDBACK

"How do I look?" girls are always asking everyone who crosses their paths, and then will listen raptly to the criticisms of greengrocers and three-year-old children. This is not always wise, since greengrocers think anything out of hair curlers is ravishing and three-year-olds tend to be bitingly critical before they've had their naps.

But still a girl needs feedback, since sometimes even the best of us will go off the deep end and become enchanted with pearlized puce eye shadow.

Who you should listen to:

—Any ex-boyfriend with whom you are now on friendly terms.

—Gay waiters in fancy restaurants, since they know everything.

—Any single girlfriend, except during the crucial period when you're on your way to a party which promises to feature several single men. Even the best of us may falter at such a moment.

—Any married girlfriend whose husband is out of town.

—Mick Jagger, if you can get hold of him.

Who you shouldn't listen to:

—Anyone remotely related to you. Even a third cousin will tell you to push the hair out of your face.

—Construction workers, who always seem to adore you at your utter frumpiest.

—Strangers on the subway. Who knows where they've been?

—Any current boyfriend, since any even vaguely negative comment he might make will be indelibly imprinted on your brain for time immemorial.

—Don Rickles.

17

Sex Tips #4—Is There Such a Thing as a Jaded Sexual Palate?

Yes. The world is riddled with bacchanalian thrill-seekers who, in their fervid, never-pausing quest to go further and deeper down heretofore unexplored, uncharted and unprecedented sexual paths, have gotten a little carried away.

WHY?

Three common American phenomena have conspired to form the jaded sexual palate: cocktail parties, television talk shows, and supermarket checkout lines.

At one time in the far distant past, cocktail parties were mere innocent skirmishes. One spoke of this and that—whether the President was an ass or not, who set fire to whose desk at which advertising agency, whether or not drugs that cured epilepsy could also get you high, etc. The only sex involved was that which was being practiced by an impetuous couple in the broom closet.

But nowadays, cocktail parties are rife with sex. The *mot juste* has been replaced by a "Can you top this?" brand of sexual repartee.

"I am thinking of having my nipples pierced," a woman with a martini in her hand will say challengingly to a man she's just met.

"Good idea," he'll say. "I just bought a new cock ring yesterday myself."

Television talk shows are equally forthcoming. No talk-show host feels his sixty minutes are complete unless forty-two of these minutes are devoted to five men "sharing" with the studio audience the fact that they truss, whip, and muzzle other consenting adult men for a living, and a pretty good living at that.

But supermarket checkout lines are the worst. I was in the A & P yesterday, waiting to pay for my meager assortment of tinned soup, yogurt and light bulbs, when my attention was arrested by the conversation of two women standing in front of me.

"Well," said the first woman (bleached eyebrows, pink acrylic pullover), "I just manipulate the clitoris with my index and third finger, and it blows my mind every time."

"Ah," said the second woman (hennaed ringlets, harem trousers), "but if you used my method, and flexed your pvc muscle, you could have seven vaginal contractions! Beat that!"

Beat what?

Sex does not like to be brought out in the open like this. A shy, retiring, sneaky, furtive sort of flower, sex shuns publicity. It wants to live a quiet, peaceful life in the gutter where it belongs.

Occasionally sex strikes an angry blow. For instance, a humiliating disease. "That'll shut them up for a while," sex mused happily as it unleashed Herpes on an unsuspecting public.

But plans, as ever, went awry, and sex was foiled again. Instead of quieting the populace, Herpes made the cover of *Time* magazine.

"Is there nothing they *won't* talk about?" sex raged, clapping an anguished hand to its forehead.

Sex is forced to come up with newer, stranger, more exotic depravities, just to get people to shut up.

WHAT EXACTLY ARE THESE NEW, STRANGE DEPRAVITIES?

It's hard to say, since newer and stranger and more depraved depravities come on the market every day, but these are the highlights so far. I am not advocating any of them. Most of them are silly, some are even dangerous. I am merely reporting.

1. *Someone tying up someone else.*

This is a popular activity, often called bondage. One may use strong cord, flexible chains, hemp, velvet ropes, licorice, shoelaces, hair ribbons, nylon stockings, belts, scarves, bandages or the ever-popular silk necktie.

One can tie the other to tables, chairs, bedposts, drainpipes, banisters, hatstands, nautilus machines, jungle gyms, piano legs, radiators, patio furniture, bus shelters, or, for that romantic touch, rose trellises.

The point of being the tie-upper is that one can playact being punishing and controlling. You have your lover at your mercy, which can be particularly attractive if same lover has been squeezing the toothpaste tube from the middle, eating the last piece of chocolate cake, or not noticing one's pretty new dress. One can vent one's pent-up anger, frustrations, and pique.

The point of being the tie-uppee is that you can feign passivity and innocence. Then, when all sorts of filthy things are being done to you, you can say to yourself, "Who, me? None of this is *my* fault! I was just minding my own business and suddenly these ropes around my wrists! I have no choice! If he wants to have his way with me I'll just have to let him! Of course, I'm not enjoying myself, not for a second. I'm just a poor helpless lamb. A poor little lamb. A poor itty-bitty lamb. A poor eensy-teensy lamb. Nothing to do with me, all this."

2. *Doing it while someone else is watching.*

Although this activity often plays a big part in many thoroughly respectable people's fantasy lives, few actually indulge.

But there are some who wrest themselves beyond the fantasy stage and hit the actual, and one wishes they hadn't bothered.

It seems that those people who most like to perform sex in public are those nobody wants to watch. One sees them prancing around all the time on ill-produced cable TV shows, and one quickly switches the channel. Possibly one sees them live, in the actual flesh, at semiprivate orgies.

The prototype male exhibitionist has a pronounced paunch, rampant hair covering his back, a vandyke beard, and gold chains (optional but preferred) festooned around the neck.

The female prototype is either much too thin or much too chubby. She has sagging breasts, thin, oily hair, and purple bruises sprinkled liberally over her body.

3. *Watching others do it.*

This is an extremely popular activity, especially among men. But watching a live performance can be profoundly disappointing and even a bit nauseating (see above). Much, much better, if one likes to watch, to go to the movies. Pornographic-movie actors are not, to be sure, an exquisite bunch, but they must be up to the reasonably attractive standards of their trade.

It is also heartening to realize that they are being paid to do this and are not simply random sleazoids.

4. *Wearing leather underwear.*

No one actually does this.

5. *Wearing rubber underwear.*

No one you'd ever want to know actually does this.

6. *Employing whips.*

For unfathomable reasons, men like to be whipped more than women do. And corporation presidents, shipping magnates, and slum landlords are alleged to prefer whipping more than electricians, locksmiths, and waiters. (Why, one hesitates to hazard a guess.)

Women who like to be whipped have often had a Catholic upbringing, which, one hears, muddles up one's pain-pleasure responses.

Whips come in all shapes and sizes, and can easily be fashioned from everyday articles found around the home. Witness how efficiently the Joan Crawford figure managed with wire clothes hangers in the movie *Mommie Dearest*.

It is never advisable to fraternize with a man who displays whips on the wall of his living room.

7. *Golden showers or water sports.*

If you know what these are, fine. If not, ask someone else. I'm not in the mood.

8. *Group sex.*

In group sex, there are endless variables: Two men with a girl. Two girls with a man. Two girls, two men. Five men, one girl. Five men, one girl and a sheep. Five men, one girl, a sheep, and a German shepherd. Five men, one girl, a sheep, a German shepherd, and a chicken. Two chickens, a sheep, and a German shepherd.

But group sex is usually limited to humans and is either of the spontaneous or nonspontaneous kind.

Spontaneous group sex occurs when everyone's had too much to drink or, more often, several Quaaludes. Complications often ensue the next morning when a very hung over group of people wake up among a large untidy pile of randomly strewn underwear and upended furniture. Usually the bathtub is full, although no one remembers using it. In fact, nobody remembers much of *anything*, but they have their suspicions.

The only thing to do in such a situation is this: Have the least hung over of the group phone a maid service for an emergency visit (at times like these, expenses be damned). Then all concerned should go for a nice brunch to a quiet, relaxed restaurant with plenty of pink lighting to neutralize green complexions. The brunch should commence with several extra-spicy Bloody Marys (doubles). Acceptable topics of conversation include the weather, the latest fall fashions, and good books one has read lately. Unacceptable topics include venereal disease, divorce laws, comparative sizes of male genitalia, and cellulite.

If one member of the group seems on the verge of collapse and keeps tearing out bits of his hair and muttering, "What have I done?" all the other members should immediately distract him by promising to chip in and buy him a condominium.

If the brunch goes *too* well, and copious amounts of Bloody Marys are consumed, the group could find itself back at square one, amidst the tangled underwear and furniture. Repeat procedure as above.

Nonspontaneous group sex is creepy, boring, and passé. Practitioners of this sport call themselves "swingers." (I ask you.) Swingers are all from the suburbs and consequently brain-addled by car pools, shopping malls, and welcome wagons. Swinger men affect furtive eyes and oozing, glutinous voices. Swinger women wear complicated hairdos and sheepish expressions.

9. *Wife-swapping*.

Just like swinging, only even more depressing.

10. *Bestiality*.

This is the sort of thing indulged in by callow farm lads and kinky Russian empresses. One may occasionally look upon an attractive Labrador retriever with speculation, but one should under no circumstances act.

11. *Sex in dangerous places.*

Dangerous may be too strong a word, since the fun lies not in risking one's life, but in the risk of getting caught. This adds a certain spice, a certain brittle gaiety, a certain heady rush of adrenalin. And this is one practice that I do approve of, if done discreetly.

You should begin gradually. Practice in places that are merely unconventional, like on the couch. On the floor. Under the kitchen table. Up against any wall. Sitting on the bathroom sink. In the shower. On the stairs.

Escalate slowly. Start doing it in the hallway of your apartment building, on your front lawn, on the roof, in the back of your car.

Then become full-fledged. Do it on other people's front lawns. Do it in other people's cars, on other people's roofs and lawns. Do it in a taxi, in a limousine, in a bus, airplane, or train. Do it in the forest. Do it on the beach. Do it in the ocean, in a swimming pool. Do it on balconies. Do it in your sister's greenhouse. Do it in art museums. Do it on stairwells in office buildings. Do it behind supermarkets. Do it on pool tables, in children's playgrounds. Do it in closets at cocktail parties. Do it in elevators. Do it in boardrooms. Do it at highway rest stops. Do it on the edge of a cliff.

When doing all this, it is a good idea to wear a voluminous skirt, which may be pulled up and down at a moment's notice. It is an even better idea to not wear underpants, but merely your stockings and garter belt. Do not fail to inform your mate of this omission. The sentence "Oh dear, I've forgotten to put on my panties again!" is guaranteed to set a man thinking along just the lines you want him to.

WHAT ABOUT SEX AND DRUGS?

Some people think drugs go with anything, and possibly they're right. But combining drugs and sex is intricate, exacting business, not to be undertaken lightly.

—*Sex and cocaine:* First you'll discuss where you want to do it.

On the bed? Or would it be more fun to do it in the shower? The shower's got a lot going for it, doesn't it? You can soap each other up. The shower. Right. Definitely. Gotta find some towels. Where the hell are the goddamned towels? Better have another snort before looking for the towels. Ah, that's better. Where were we? Oh, right, sex. Shower. Before we do it, I just want to tell you one thing. Back when I was three years old (twenty-minute story ensues).

Don't you think it's time for another little one? Just a line? Ah, that's better, but I think I'm getting a little wired. Do you have any Valium? You don't? Oh, God. If I had known you didn't have any Valium I wouldn't have . . . No, I'm *not* saying it's your fault, really I'm not. It's just that . . . but . . . uh huh . . . uh huh . . . right . . . uh huh . . . sure . . . no . . . uh huh . . . um . . . that's just exactly . . . oh . . . uh huh . . . uh huh . . . then what happened?

What did you say, just that last thing? I was grinding my teeth too hard to hear you. Oh, right, the shower. Well, it's not that I don't want to exactly, but I have to go out now. For a walk or something. No, it's nothing. I just feel a little nervous. Maybe if we went for a drink . . . What? It's *five* A.M.? You're kidding, right?

And that will be that. Some say that they rub cocaine on the penis to anesthetize it and give it a little staying power. This is a bad waste of good cocaine. Men on cocaine do not come too quickly. Often they do not come at all.

—*Sex and marijuana:* This is a wonderful combination if you think the sun rises and sets on your fellow and you are convinced he feels the same about you. But if there is even the soupçon of a doubt in either department, things could bend sinister.

"Why is he taking off his clothes in such a strange manner?" you'll think to yourself. "He's left his socks on."

"You've left your socks on," you'll tell him.

"Ha ha ha, so I have," he'll chuckle.

You won't like that chuckle. It will have a strange, brittle ring, if you ask you. The guy probably doesn't like you. He's just going through the motions.

"Why are you looking at me like that?" he'll say.

"What are you talking about?"

"You're giving me this strange, faraway look."

"I am not. You're just paranoid."

"No, I'm not."

"Yes you are."

"Are what?"

"Are what what?"

"What are we talking about?"

"It was socks, wasn't it?"

"Was it?"

"Was what?"

"What what?"

"Jesus, that was dynamite shit."

"God, yes, I'm really stoned."

"Me too."

You'll wonder if he's lying. He'll wonder if you're lying. You'll wonder if he's wondering if you're lying. He'll wonder the same. Fleeting doubts will become fixed and motionless. You'll both fall asleep.

—*Sex and psychedelics:* This is never recommended, for the simple reason that your partner could turn into a two-headed, seven-foot-long lizard if you take your eyes off him for a second. Even if you don't.

—*Sex and Quaaludes:* Sex on Quaaludes is everything that is wild, uninhibited, wanton, and shameless. You'll say anything, do anything. It will be exactly the sort of tryst the memories of which would still bring a gleam to your eye fifty years from now when you're tooling around the old-age home in your motorized wheelchair.

Trouble is, by the next morning, you will have forgotten everything.

—*Sex and speed:* If you relish the idea of four hours of tireless fucking and neither of you actually coming, this is the drug for you.

—*Sex and alcohol:* Use alcohol sparingly. No more than a bottle of wine between you and two margaritas each. A drunken man is a lust-crazed beast with a glittering, licentious eye. He will pay you all sorts of compliments and tell you all the vile yet wonderful acts he wishes to perpetrate on your body. Then he will fall asleep on top of you before he actually gets it in.

WITH ALL THIS NEW, FREE SEXUALITY, ARE IMPOTENCE AND PREMATURE EJACULATION ON THE DECLINE?

No, but they're not on the rise either.

How Can We Cure Impotence and Premature Ejaculation?

First-night impotence is only the jitters and needn't worry you. Even second-night impotence is no cause for alarm. But if we're talking prolonged, chronic impotence, chances are you have a guilty man in your arms.

The most common cause of impotence in men is marriage to other women. The penis knows its Ten Commandments, and this is its own, quirky way of slapping its owner's hand.

"Don't touch!" the penis says.

"But I want to!" pleads the man.

"I don't care," says the penis primly. "It's just not done, old sport. You've got that nice little woman waiting for you at home."

"Just this once, now I've gotten this far?" the man asks wistfully.

"No," says the penis. "If I let you this time, then you'll want just one more time, and one more time after that, and pretty soon we won't know where we are."

"I know where I wish *you* were," says the man bitterly.

"Well, I'm not going there. It's just not right. Now quit this nonsense and let's go home."

He may, of course, *not* be married, just living with someone. Or maybe it's that you're married. To his best friend. Or his brother. Or maybe his best friend has a crush on you. Or maybe he's mother-fixated. Who knows?

All you know for sure is that it's out of your hands. A man with heavy impotence problems is not your problem.

You can't cure him. Oh, you can be loving and understanding and try every fellatio trick known to woman, but if nothing works, don't take it personally. If you do, *you'll* start feeling guilty, thinking you must be doing something wrong, or that you're just not attractive enough. This is not true, since no man goes to bed with a woman he isn't attracted to unless she pays him a lot of money.

If you love him, send him to a shrink or make an appointment for the two of you with a sex therapist who does not advertise in the classified section of *Screw* magazine.

Or, just on a long shot, you could say, "Gee, it's great to see you darling. But I'm not going to let you fuck me today, no matter what."

Premature ejaculation has many causes, the most prominent of which is anger.

"The hell with her!" a man's subconscious is saying, "Why should I let *her* have any pleasure. I'll just get my rocks off and leave her hanging!"

A man usually doesn't realize any of this. All he knows is he can't control himself and he's getting these awful anxiety attacks about it.

One way to surmount this problem is to pick a fight with him. Start anywhere. He leaves his hair all over the bathroom sink. He's a lousy tipper. Whatever. If you play it right, you can escalate the fight out of all proportion until you get him screaming and frothing at the mouth. He may then actually tell you what's really bothering him. But even if he doesn't, you should be in for some terrific sex.

Always remember that guilt and anger are the heavies in nearly everyone's life, and can spoil a woman's pleasure just as thoroughly as a man's.

DOES A MAN'S SIZE HAVE ANYTHING TO DO WITH A WOMAN'S PLEASURE?

Stop any girl on the street and ask her if she cares if a man is well hung, and she will look at you aghast.

"Of course not," she'll say, "it's not what you've got, it's how you use it. It's not the meat, it's the motion."

But get a group of girls together around closing time at some sleazy joint with plenty of Hank Williams on the jukebox, and the girls will come clean.

"Well, I have to admit it," said Cleo recently at some sleazy joint at 2 A.M., "but I like big ones. Not huge or anything, but, you know, good size."

"What's good size?" wondered Marta, "six inches?"

"Eight," Cleo said dreamily, "or nine. After nine it gets problematical."

"And after ten it hurts," said Rita.

"Well, I don't think it matters at all if you love him," said Kate sweetly.

"We have here our token newlywed," said Cleo.

"Well, darlin'," said Rita, "it doesn't exactly *matter*, it's just nice when they're big, that's all. Pleasant to look at. Any girl who pretends otherwise is just working overtime on bein' one of them total women. Or else she's a social worker. But it doesn't actually *matter*, when you get right down to it. One of my husbands had this itty-bitty cock, and that man still to this very day drives me insane with lust. If he walked in here right now, I'd be on him like a duck on a junebug."

We pondered this for a while. Then Kate spoke.

"Thick ones are always nice," she said.

"I like a thick one myself," said Marta.

"Who doesn't?" said Cleo. "I will now tell you a little-known fact, not to be repeated beyond these four walls."

We all leaned forward, agog.

"We only have nerve endings in the first three inches of our vaginas," Cleo said, "beyond that, we feel nothing, *nada*, zip."

There was a general uproar. Kate upset her drink, Rita called for a double tequila. Marta fell backward in her chair. I dropped my tape recorder.

This was a stunning blow.

"I don't believe it for a minute," said Kate.

"Utterly ridiculous," said Marta.

"A barefaced lie," said Rita.

"God's truth," said Cleo.

This called for a bit more pondering.

"So then why," said I, "do we care how big they are? If what you say is true, three inches should do us just fine."

"Yes and no," said Cleo. "What good do big tits do? None. But some men crave them."

"*Most* men," said Marta, a bit sadly.

"Well," said Cleo, "it's the same thing, is all."

The same, yet different.

18

Travel Tips

It is always a good idea to take a little trip, since the chances of having a good time while on the road are enhanced by probably 451 percent. A girl gadding about is (a) footloose and fancy free, (b) able to lie about her age, roots, name, profession, marital status and mental health without anyone finding out, and (c) able to carry on in such a way and with such fellows as would cause many a raised eyebrow and sarcastic comment from her friends at home.

Travel whenever you're feeling like a dried-up old toad. It is a scientific fact that when a woman is feeling like a dried-up old toad, even one night in another town, especially a smallish town down south or out west, will transform her into a sparkling, wit-infested, moist and magical femme fatale with fatal and mysterious charm.

Since I need this kind of fix more than I like to think, I have become somewhat of an expert in the field of intercontinental travel with trouble-making intent. Here are some pointers:

1. *Never go to Boston.* Boston is a singularly horrific city, full

of surly weirdos with scraggly beards and terrible manners. Plus you will probably die, since Bostonians drive very stupidly and all the road signs are specifically designed to hopelessly scramble the brains of anyone needing to know the way. If you don't die, you will get lost—even people who actually live in Boston (unappealing college students) can never find the way to the corner.

Even New Jersey is better than Boston. Even Cleveland, even Miami Beach. Anywhere.

2. *Never pack more than you can comfortably carry.*

One should always be prepared to vanish at the drop of a hat. Perhaps that wise, picturesque goat-roper suddenly reveals himself to be a homicidal maniac. Possibly the girlfriend of that sweet, witty architect arrives prematurely from Europe. Jealous wives could come careening dangerously along in pickup trucks.

You should be able to pack your things and be out of your motel in approximately three seconds flat, or before the homicidal maniac can get there with a shotgun, whichever comes first.

Besides these farfetched eventualities, carrying heavy bags will put you inevitably in a foul temper. All you need is:

Toothbrush, shampoo, minimal toiletries.

Several pairs of stockings, two garter belts, a couple of lacy bras, a silk slip, a gorgeous satin robe.

White dress, white trousers, several white shirts.

Black dress, black trousers, two black shirts.

Black or red heels.

White sneakers.

(Take colored clothes if you must, but you will then be less striking and suffer coordination problems.)

Fur coat or bathing suit, depending on season.

Birth control.

A heavy blunt instrument.

3. *Never pack easy-care fabrics or pantyhose in little eggs.*

People are always telling you to do this, but staring at wrinkle-free polyester will only make you sad. Take your most beautifully cut clothes. Your sexiest shoes.

If your clothes get wrinkled, just steam them in the bathroom. What, after all, are those boiling hot showers in Holiday Inns for?

4. *When going to county fairs, do not eschew cute shoes.*

I shall never, as long as I live, forget the time when Cleo and I were at the Washington County Fair in Rhode Island and came upon the dreamiest man in creation. He was, I believe, something called a "soundman." Cleo and I went into furious competition, and the soundman was bedazzled and bemused. He couldn't seem to make up his mind, until he espied Cleo's totally impractical pink heels. I, in my sadly infinite wisdom, had decided on old sneakers since it was muddy.

5. *Make sure you know how to dance.*

In that big, wide country out there, not all people discuss the films they've seen lately or who's been lunching with whom at the Russian Tea Room. This may seem impossible, but it's true. What Americans mainly do is dance. And they actually know how to, which is more than we can say for residents of New York and Los Angeles, where they dance ten feet apart, glazed eyes staring out into space.

The folks at, say, the Ramada Inn in Santa Fe (where a good friend of mine met her husband) dance close, dance slow, dance sexy. It will not hurt you at all to learn the rudiments of the two-step. When a cowboy asks you to dance, he may well say Please, and call you Ma'am. Do not be misled into thinking his courtliness means he is an insipid, tentative lover. Quite the contrary.

6. *Rent a car whenever possible, FM radio desirable.*

There is nothing better for the psyche than cruising down strange highways at dawn with the windows rolled down and the radio blasting "Bad Moon Rising." A woman I know found Zen truth this way.

7. *Beware of men on airplanes.*

The minute a man reaches 30,000 feet, he becomes immediately consumed by distasteful sexual fantasies which involve doing uncomfortable things in those tiny toilets. These men should not be encouraged, their fantasies are sadly low-rent and unimaginative. Affect an aloof, cool demeanor as soon as any man tries to draw you out. Unless, of course, he's the pilot.

8. *Think twice about men on trains.*

Amorous men on trains may be in the throes of a Nick and Nora Charles fantasy, since most of the *Thin Man* movies end up with N & N falling on each other in one of those luxuriant Pullman compartments while Asta looks askance. This sort of man could be amusing.

But then again, the guy could just have read *Fear of Flying* and be entertaining ideas of zipless fucks, much less appealing.

9. *Never travel on a bus unless you have to.*

This defeats the whole purpose of traveling, since you will not have a good time. Also, all cute men on buses are ex-convicts and usually bigamists.

10. *Don't go out of your way to meet men.*

The moment a stranger arrives in town she exudes enough come-hither vibes to bring the entire male population of Peoria to its knees, so be careful. No indiscriminate batting of eyelashes, no randomly directed inviting smiles, or you'll be stampeded by rampaging men, many of whom may be unattractive.

So peruse carefully and circumspectly, until you see exactly the one you want. Then simply ask for a light.

11. *Whenever possible, travel with a friend.*

It's sometimes intimidating to walk into strange nightclubs alone, and it's always nice to have someone along to read the road map.

And you need someone to talk to, so you can ask, "So? What do you think? Is he dumb, or just unsophisticated? I'll walk past him now, you see if he looks. But what should I say to him? Is he looking now? Do you think he's married? Hey, wait a minute, how about that one? Do these shoes go with this dress? Can I borrow your mascara?"

This friend should be female, if possible, or things could get complicated. And this female friend should preferably like a different type of man than you do, or things could get strained. If things *do* get strained, remember that a good friend is harder to find than a cute man.

12. *Do not automatically assume that farmers are stupid.*

13. *Do not automatically assume that farmers are romantic and deep.*

14. *Do not decide to "go native."*

There is something inherently unpleasant about a sophisticated girl from Chicago showing up at a kicker bar in Austin, Texas, in a ten-gallon hat and embroidered cowboy boots.

15. *Keep away from men who wear guns.*

16. *Think carefully before letting a strange man buy you a drink at a bar.*

In some parts of the country, they still think this means you're definitely going to sleep with them.

17. *And absolutely under no circumstances accept drinks from more than one man at a bar.* A brawl is inevitable.

18. *Beware of random sex.*

When you're out of town, even the most fleeting liaison has an alarming tendency to turn into a full-fledged romance, sometimes even marriage. No one knows why this is. You could end up with astronomical phone bills, you could end up having to move permanently to Utah. Be forewarned.

19. *Make sure to travel when brokenhearted.*

19

How to Cure a Broken Heart

"If heartaches were commercials, we'd all be on TV."
—JOHN PRINE

COSMIC PROLOGUE

"Goddamned butter," Rita sobbed as she threw her toast across the room. The butter had been offensively solid, which was exactly more than Rita could take at the moment.

The night before, her boyfriend had appeared at her door, let himself in with his key, and stared at her mournfully.

"I'm thinking of getting married," he said.

Rita perked up, but then she took a careful look at his face.

"To whom?" she said, grammatically correct to the end.

"This dancer I met three weeks ago," he said.

Thus the far-flung toast.

Next thing she knew, Rita was in her rusty old Cadillac, driving straight into the desert. She didn't stop until she got to the Space-Age Motel on Interstate 25, somewhere around Gila Bend, Arizona. She checked in.

Rita is a big, strong Texas girl, smart and sassy, always ready for anything. And yet she now had serious trouble walking the couple of yards across the parking lot to the Space-Age Cafe, an adjunct to the Space-Age Motel.

She sat down at the gold-flecked Formica booth and ordered grits, eggs, and coffee. A vague feeling of peace stole over her as she contemplated bloodcurdling revenge.

"That disgusting, vile, depraved son of a scumbag," Rita mused about the man she loved. "I'll cut his heart out with an ax. I'll amputate his feet with a buzzsaw."

A man sat down at her table, uninvited.

He wore a green J.C. Penney work suit, several pens stuck out of his perma-press shirt pocket. His face was round and meek, his eyes vague behind wire-rimmed glasses.

"You remind me of my daughter," the man said, motioning to the waitress for some coffee. "My daughter just ran away from her husband. Took her mother's car. What she had in mind was driving that car right out to California and clear into the ocean. Her own mother's car. You on the run, hon?"

Rita stared, the grits dropping off her fork. "You might say," she said.

"Thought so," he said, "you got the earmarks of a bad love affair all over you. Look at the way you're sitting, shoulders all hunched up like that. Bad for your posture, you know. Look at those grits dribbling all over your chin.

"But lemme tell you about love," he continued.

"Here it comes," thought Rita.

"Love," said the man firmly. "You never get anywhere until you figure out the difference between passion and compassion. Love affairs that begin in passion burn themselves out real quick, like blue stars. You gotta watch out for them, hon, they can burn you up too.

"But then there's the love affairs that begin in compassion, those are the ones you want to find. They just build and build into real passion and then, well, then it's like you can just drive into the sky, right up into and right past those blue stars. You want some more coffee or what?"

The man went off somewhere, possibly out to a waiting spaceship. Rita sat and digested his words and her breakfast. Then he reappeared.

"Hon," he said, "I just want you to know your breakfast is taken care of. Least I could do, the way you remind me of my daughter and all." He walked away, came back, waggled his finger at her. "Now you remember, don't retaliate. I know you want to. But those things have a habit of boomeranging right back at you. Leave it alone. You'll be all right. You'll be just fine."

Back in the motel room she was beginning to call home, Rita unearthed a poetry book, flipped idly through it. Some words sprang out at her, clamoring for attention.

"The beauty of men never disappears," the book proclaimed, "but drives a blue car through the stars."

Rita looked around nervously, kind of expecting Rod Serling to emerge from behind the shower curtain.

The next day Rita was driving along in the blistering heat of Route 62, when she suddenly felt the need to stop the car and stare aimlessly at cactus.

A passing police car screeched to a halt ten yards from her, a state trooper got out.

"How ya doin', darlin'?" he asked conversationally.

"Just fine," Rita said.

"I bet you're not just fine," the trooper answered, taking his revolver out of its holster. He aimed the gun skyward and fired three times. The shots jolted Rita's brain, realigning its cells.

"You'll be okay now," he said. "Just a touch of desert rapture."

"So listen, sugar," Rita said to me later that month, "if you'll just let them, people will be there when you need them. Heartbreak is horrible, but the dancing girls will always just keep on dancing."

"What dancing girls?" I asked, since I am not a Texan.

When treating yourself for heartbreak, make sure you really have it. All too often, a girl will fully believe her heart is broken when she is simply suffering from severe ego perforation.

To find out, take this simple quiz:

1. When I cry my eyes out at night, the thing that bothers me most is:

(a) The fact that he's got this new, incredibly blond floozy whom he's squiring all over town and it hasn't even been two weeks yet.

(b) The realization that never again will someone whose hair smells exactly like fresh lima beans be waking me in the middle of the night for a quick one.

2. When I'm lying in the bathtub constructing fantasy conversations with him, these conversations usually involve:

(a) Me explaining sweetly how his penis is too small anyway.

(b) The two of us chatting jauntily about how silly we've been to think we could live without each other.

3. When I see happy couples on the street, I want to

(a) Puke my guts out.

(b) Puke my guts out.

If you answered (a) to the above questions, you're probably just suffering from rejection, and also miffed. Simple rejection, when your feelings aren't seriously engaged, is certainly not pleasant, but you'll get over it the minute you have a minute.

But if your answers were predominantly (b), you are suffering from clinical heartbreak and must take serious measures.

Clinical heartbreak is comprised of various elements which all blend together into one turbulent and devastating alloy. We shall take these elements one by one and examine them.

HEARTBREAK ELEMENT #1—LOSS OF REALITY

When you spend most of your time with another person, you create your own little world, a custom-made planet built for two. A planet encased in a climate-controlled bubble, effectively barricaded from the malicious elements of the outside world. The longer you stay in the planetary bubble, the more vegetation grows, the more curtains are hung in the windows, the more homey and cozy it becomes.

The Gary-and-Sue planet, if you will. With Gary-and-Sue jokes that no one else understands, Gary-and-Sue experiences that no one else knows about, Gary-and-Sue sex games that nobody better *ever* know about. Gary-and-Sue favorite books. Gary-and-Sue favorite tapes. Gary-and-Sue exercise routines. Gary-and-Sue sporting events. Gary-and-Sue pregnancy scares. Gary-and-Sue plate-smashing marathons.

When Gary-and-Sue break up, it's as though Darth Vader located their innocent little planet in his sights and smashed it to smithereens, turning it to random clouds of aimless asteroids.

And Gary and Sue, who may have despised each other at the time of the breakup, will nonetheless find themselves wandering about their lives trying to create order among the asteroids which once comprised their world.

Sue, browsing in an antique shop, will find one of those funny old matchboxes that Gary used to crave, and she will have her money out of her wallet before the sad realization hits. Those funny little matchboxes have no place in her life anymore! Sue is filled with panic, confusion. If she's not looking for matchboxes, what *is* she looking for? Maybe she should just buy this one, just this once, and send it to Gary. . . . No! What could she be thinking? He is the scum of the earth! So Sue just wanders out of the antique shop, tries to figure out if she wants to turn right or left, and bursts into tears.

Meanwhile Gary, feeling a bit peckish one evening, decides to treat himself to a nice fancy dinner. Where to go? He can't go to Mickey's, since that's where Sue ate too much chocolate mousse and threw up all over the maitre d'. How about the Odeon? Nah, that's where they took Sue's mother when they were trying to squeeze a down payment for a summer house out of the old bird. La Gamelle? No, Sue always craved the bartender, he doesn't want to look at that bartender's face right now. The Frog and Peach? Maybe. Sue always hated it. That's what he'll do, now that he's free as a breeze, he'll go to The Frog and Peach. And he does. But when he gets there, he feels guilty. Guilty, for chrissakes! He keeps seeing why Sue hated this phony place full of phony waiters and phony coat-check girls and phony margaritas. Sue would absolutely laugh her throaty little laugh at the way the wine steward called the Moët 66 "loquacious." So Gary slinks out, Sue's throaty little laugh echoing in his brain, back to his sudden bachelor pad, where even the goddamned toothpaste tube reminds him of goddamned Sue.

HEARTBREAK ELEMENT #2— MISPLACEMENT OF SELF

One often, especially if one is a woman and therefore taught almost from birth to do this, identifies oneself with the object of one's affections. If your husband is the president of a big deal corporation, then you are the president of a big deal corporation's wife and therefore pretty hot stuff. If you are a rock star's girlfriend, you are automatically a reigning queen of hipness.

When the relationship is torn asunder, you don't know who you are, which leads to feelings of abandonment, worthlessness, and other grisly sentiments. Your self-esteem goes into hiding and must be carefully coaxed to reemerge.

HEARTBREAK ELEMENT #3—FEAR

Will you ever find another man? Are you going to die cold and miserable and lonely? There are no men out there anymore, right? All your friends say that all men are either gay or married, and they're probably right. So what are you going to do? Who's going to love you? You're not so special, are you? And you're certainly not as young as you used to be. Do all men only want nineteen-year-olds? What if you're too smart? What if you're too stupid? What if you have bad breath and that's why he left you? If he left you, you must be unlovable, right? How are you going to spend tomorrow night? How about the night after that? What if you never again meet anyone? What if you never again get laid?

HEARTBREAK ELEMENT #4—SADNESS

It's sad stuff, losing someone you once loved, no matter how good the reason, no matter how justified you are, no matter what.

Depressing business, heartbreak, no picnic no matter how you look at it.

But never fear, you can cure yourself if you feel like it. Follow these handy instructions.

RAVE, MOAN, SCREAM, WAIL AND SOB

Back in say, 1807, heartbreak was treated with the respect it deserves. Women whose hearts were broken went into an immediate decline and spent months in bed having vinaigrette pressed to their noses and laudanum poured down their throats. Anxious relatives hovered about the heartbreak victim's bedside, hoping she wouldn't die. Sometimes she did.

But now tell someone your heart is broken and she'll tell you to buy a new hat. This attitude, free and breezy as it may be, is ridiculous. Heartbreak is as traumatic to body and soul as major surgery, and even if you were to buy fifty new hats, even fifty new hats with fetching little veils, you would still feel that life is a hollow, horrible joke. (A Valentino ballgown—*that* might have a chance of perking you up. Or possibly a set of perfectly matched emerald earrings could bring a wan smile to your lips.)

So pay no mind to hat theories and let yourself suffer profusely. Don't pretend to be fine.

I knew a fellow once who pretended that his broken heart didn't exist. Fellow named David.

"Ha ha ha," David chortled loudly when his wife of eight years decided she couldn't stand the sight of him.

"Ha ha ha," David chortled endlessly. "What do I care? She can go to hell for all she means to me. She can take her pick of slow boats to China. She can go and marry Robert Redford and I won't turn a hair, now that I've got you."

"You" was me, and I had been dating him for three weeks when I couldn't help noticing that David seemed to have temper tantrums if he ordered lemon meringue pie and the waiter said there wasn't any. Once, while we were driving down Fifth Avenue, David jumped out of his car and began physically assaulting a taxi driver who had cut him off at the light.

David didn't mind in the least when I called the whole thing off. "Ha ha," he giggled, "there will be others."

And there were. There was Mona, and Judy, and Betsy, and Ruth, and Phoebe, and Jill.

"How's Jill?" I said to David recently.

"Ah, Jill," David said. "Lovely girl. Terrific person. But, I don't know, something's missing. I'm just not in love. Terribly sweet girl, Jill. Did I tell you that the other night I met a girl who is *so* wonderful it is not to be believed? Cleo. She has everything. Looks, wit, glamour . . ."

Cleo? Oh no, it couldn't be.

"Sure," said my buddy Cleo. "I met David a couple of weeks ago. Cute fellow. I liked him a lot until he threw a saltshaker at a waiter because there was no lemon meringue pie. And then he asks me to go to Jamaica for a month. What's the story with this guy?"

I'm going to make a wild accusation here: David never got over his wife's leaving him. He took all his pain and rage and buried it, gave it the cold shoulder and refused to let it manifest itself. But pain and rage don't take kindly to being ignored, and clamor for release, even inappropriate release. Thus we have saltshakers hurled at hapless waiters.

And although David may babble on at excruciating length on the subject of finding the woman of his dreams, he is very efficiently avoiding this eventuality by acting like a lunatic. Someone once called this syndrome "fear of intimacy," which simply translated means "Hi there, don't get close to me, I don't want to get hurt again."

The world is becoming increasingly populated with this variety of walking wounded. Most of them are men, for, as Richard Pryor once said, "when a woman's heart is broken, she cries and shit. But men don't cry, they take a walk and get run over by a truck. Don't even see it." But we women, in our constant struggle for equality, are now aping this stiff-upper-lip routine, with much the same results.

So feel free to have hysterics. Collapse into heaps. Speak in sepulchral whispers, go into deep mourning, cry your eyes out. When people ask how you are, tell them. Howl. Throw things. Buy a punching bag and use it. Get drunk and pass out.

SHAMELESSLY RELY ON YOUR BEST FRIEND

Call her and tell her you don't care if she's supposed to be accepting the Nobel Peace Prize that day, you're on your way over in a taxi and she'd better keep her priorities in order. When you get there, station yourself on her sofa and have her bring you cups of tea and cute little bonbons. Make her tell you jokes. If she gets cranky, remind her of the time she broke up with Herb and camped out on your sofa for three months.

CALL A MAID SERVICE

Tell them to send someone over immediately, preferably a gay man. Gay men, even those you've never met before, are notoriously effective for nursing a girl through a broken heart. They've been there. They care.

You and this gay man should then bundle each and every bit of evidence of your ex-lover which happens to be lurking about into one or two huge trash bags. Do not neglect the pillow where his head once nestled. Don't decide to save that frayed sock from happier days. When each emotionally laden item is assembled, throw the whole lot out the window, trying to avoid any innocent passerby, even if the top of his head reminds you of the wart you used to call your lover.

READ MURDER MYSTERIES INCESSANTLY

Especially English ones, which are a sublime blend of coziness and bloodshed, a perfect balm for shattered nerves.

GET A HAIRCUT

A brilliant, expensive, incredibly flattering haircut will put you well on the road to recovery.

PICTURE YOUR EX-LOVER IN A TUTU

You're supposed to do this, I read it in a book somewhere. If you can conjure up the image of him draped in pink frills and pirouetting onstage at a large charity benefit, your love will begin to wane.

Or, if you prefer it, picture him gaining seventy-five pounds. Or wearing a gold medallion around his neck and his shirt open to the waist while he sings "My Way." Or sporting Gucci loafers and a bandana around his head.

Do Not Call Him, Do Not Try to See Him, Never Fuck Him

The first thing a child learns in life is to run to her nearest and dearest when she is hurt.

"Daddeee!!!" a little girl will immediately scream when a bee bites her on the nose. Daddy, the little girl knows, will make it all better, will take the hurt away, will smash that bloody bee to bits.

We may now be grownups but, in this instance at least, nobody ever grows up. We still want the one we love the most to kiss it and make it better.

This leads to unfortunate situations, like the heartbreak victim calling the actual heartbreaker at 3 A.M. for a little chat, saying appalling things like "Harry? It's me. Did I wake you? Are you sure? Well listen, could you just talk to me for a minute? I can't sleep. I don't know what to do. Yes, I tried warm milk. No, I don't have any Valium. Maybe if you could just come over, just this once, and just hold me for a minute, you could make me feel better. Oh, I see, you have someone there. No, you do, I can tell by your voice. Well, why won't you come over then? Well, I don't care if it doesn't make any sense. Oh, you will? Are you sure it isn't too much trouble? Ten minutes? Surely it won't really take you ten minutes?"

And Harry, feeling guilty, trots dutifully over, holds her for a minute, and makes it all worse.

The proper time to call Harry at 3 A.M. is after you've got over him, after you've become fast friends instead of rancid lovers, and you've got new problems to deal with. If another man is doing you wrong, then having good old Harry come by to hold your hand is just fine. But never, ever, when Harry is the one doing the hurting. It isn't seemly, it isn't smart and, although it may turn out beautifully in the movies, it doesn't work in real life.

If you've tried warm milk, and you don't have any Valium, then by all means call someone and demand immediate comforting. Anybody but Harry.

And, although you may not want to go to the trouble of actually avoiding him, do not seek Harry out. Do not go to a boring party just because you know he'll be there. Do not take a detour on your way to the grocery store so that you just happen to be walking past his door. This takes enormous courage, but it's worth it, for two reasons.

1. There is always the possibility that you and Harry will get back together again. This is not a hope you should nurse, so let us just state it quickly and forget it, since nursing hopes just prolongs agony. But if you are going to get back together again, it's not going to happen if you follow him around like a stricken puppy. The stricken-puppy approach is fine for a small Pomeranian, but seems to elicit nothing but contempt when practiced by humans. Harry will miss you a lot more if you're not there.

2. If you don't get back together again, cold turkey is the only way. The reason you two were together in the first place is that you grew addicted to each other. You grew to crave each other, couldn't get enough of each other.

Especially sexually. Which is why you must never fuck him just for old time's sake or with the mistaken idea that he won't be able to live without you once you fall into bed again. Again, that stuff only happens in movies.

A sexual addiction is stronger than a heroin habit. To fuck is to get a fix. To get a fix is to be right back where you started, at the very beginning of the old heartbreak trail.

Don't even masturbate with him in mind. Replaying your greatest hits while playing with yourself will keep you firmly on the hook. Fantasize about Nick Nolte or, if you're some kind of weirdo, Tom Selleck.

TAKE THE COUNTRY-AND-WESTERN SAD SONG CURE

Ever been driving down the highway and seen a truck driver driving along with tears streaming down his face?

The trucker is not deranged. He's just heard a particularly sad Willie Nelson song on his radio and succumbed to the great Country-and-Western Catharsis.

Every single C-and-W song is about being heartbroken, except for the ones about how good old boys should just stay drunk and rowdy at all times, which I guess are just a different variety of heartbreak song. If you can listen to them in a bar accompanied by several margaritas and other assorted sobbing souls, so much the better. After taking a painstaking poll, I have come up with the ten greatest Country-and-Western songs to cure heartbreak.

Song	*Best Version Sung by*
1. Misery and Gin	Merle Haggard
2. Honky-Tonk Angels	Kitty Wells
3. The Race Is On	George Jones
4. I Fall to Pieces	Patsy Cline
5. The Last Thing I Needed the First Thing This Morning Was to Have You Walk Out On Me	Willie Nelson
6. Blue Umbrella	John Prine
7. Faded Love	Willie Nelson and Ray Price
8. Lovesick Blues	Hank Williams
9. Your Cheatin' Heart	Hank Williams
10. I'm So Lonesome I Could Cry	Hank Williams

LEAVE TOWN

This is essential for the heartbroken girl who can finally bring herself to move. Depending on the kindness of strangers, as we have shown in the Cosmic Prologue at the beginning of this chapter, can reap bountiful rewards. And there is nothing like hitting the road to give you a new perspective, not to mention as many new love interests as you feel like having.

Remember, we dancing girls are honor bound to keep on dancing.